Informatics in Primary Care

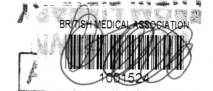

Springer Science+Business Media, LLC

Informatics in Primary Care

Strategies in Information Management for the Healthcare Provider

Thomas E. Norris, M.D.
School of Medicine and UW Physicians Network, University of Washington, Seattle, Washington USA

Sherrilynne S. Fuller, Ph.D.
School of Medicine and Information School, University of Washington, Seattle, Washington USA

Harold I. Goldberg, M.D.
School of Medicine, University of Washington, Seattle, Washington USA

Peter Tarczy-Hornoch, M.D.
School of Medicine, University of Washington, Seattle, Washington USA

Editors

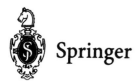

Springer

Thomas E. Norris, M.D.
Associate Dean, University of Washington
    School of Medicine
Executive Director and Medical Executive,
    University of Washington Physicians
    Network
Professor of Family Medicine
Adjunct Professor of Medicine,
    Biomedical Informatics, and
    Health Services
Box 356340
Seattle, WA 98195
USA
tnorris@u.washington.edu

Harold I. Goldberg, M.D.
Associate Professor of Medicine
Box 359780
University of Washington School of
    Medicine
Seattle, WA 98195
USA
hig@u.washington.edu

Sherrilynne S. Fuller, Ph.D.
Professor
Division of Biomedical and
    Health Informatics and Information
    School
Box 357155
University of Washington School of
    Medicine
Seattle, WA 98195
USA
sfuller@u.washington.edu

Peter Tarczy-Hornoch, M.D.
Associate Professor and Division Head,
    Biomedical and Health Informatics,
    Department of Medical Education
and
Associate Professor, Division of
    Neonatology, Department of Pediatrics
Box 356320
University of Washington
Seattle, WA 98195
USA
pth@u.washington.edu

Library of Congress Cataloging-in-Publication Data
Informatics in primary care : strategies in information management for the healthcare provider /
editors, Thomas E. Norris [et al.].
        p.   cm.
    Includes bibliographical references and index.
    ISBN 978-0-387-95333-5   ISBN 978-1-4613-0069-4 (eBook)
    DOI 10.1007/978-1-4613-0069-4
        1. Medical informatics.   2. Primary care (Medicine)   I. Norris, Thomas E.
    R858 J535   2002
    610′.285—dc21   2001042963

Printed on acid-free paper.

Production managed by MaryAnn Brickner; manufacturing supervised by Jacqui Ashri.
Typeset by Impressions Book and Journal Services, Inc., Madison, WI.

9 8 7 6 5 4 3 2 1

ISBN 978-0-387-95333-5

Preface

Informatics, the study of the science of information and related disciplines, is being increasingly applied to medicine and healthcare. Medical schools are developing departments, divisions, and sections of medical (or biomedical) informatics, and curricula are being created for medical students and residents. For many practicing physicians, questions such as "What is informatics?" and "Why is informatics important in medicine?" are becoming commonplace. Further, once these basics are understood, many physicians seek more complete information about this new "basic science."

The goal of this book is to provide primary care physicians with a practical introductory understanding of medical informatics, focusing on areas of importance in primary care. Additionally, we seek to present clinical contexts in which some of the various applications of medical informatics can be applied.

The book begins with an overview of medical informatics, based on the interaction (interface) between the patient and the primary care physician. Next, we study how this interaction can be documented with electronic medical records, and how information on laboratory data and imaging, originating from other electronic sources, can be integrated into the electronic medical record. We then cover several areas that concern the content of the information used in primary care. Areas of focus include evidence-based medicine, decision support, knowledge resources, and patient education. Finally, this book concludes with five chapters concerning practical aspects of primary care informatics: workflow, privacy and security, electronic billing, reporting and analysis, and telecommunications.

Family physicians, internists, and pediatricians will find this book useful in understanding the rapidly growing field of medical informatics. Medical students and residents will also find that the broad scope of this volume provides a useful overview. Though the focus of the book is on primary care other specialty healthcare providers will find it useful as a basic introduction to the discipline. Other primary health care students and providers, including nurses, physician assistants, and pharmacists, will find this a useful compendium of cases coupled with informatics interventions.

Some have said that the skillful management of huge quantities of information characterizes the art and practice of medicine. The task of turning that information into knowledge that can be used to improve the health of patients is the job of the physician. The study of informatics and the use of the tools of this new science have the potential to improve the healthcare and outcomes of those for whom care is provided.

Contents

Contributors

Editors

(also authored chapters)

Thomas E. Norris, M.D.
Department of Family Medicine
University of Washington
Seattle, Washington, USA

Sherrilynne S. Fuller, Ph.D.
Department of Medical Education,
Division Biomedical and Health Infor-
matics
University of Washington
Seattle, Washington, USA

Harold I. Goldberg, M.D.
Department of Medicine
University of Washington
Seattle, Washington, USA

Peter Tarczy-Hornoch, M.D.
Department of Pediatrics, Division of
Neonatology
Department of Medical Education,
Division Biomedical and Health Infor-
matics
University of Washington
Seattle, Washington, USA

Chapter Authors

(who are not editors)

Lydia Bartholomew, M.D.
Department of Family Medicine
University of Washington
Seattle, Washington, USA

David Chou, M.D.
Department of Laboratory Medicine
University of Washington
Seattle, Washington, USA

Paul D. Clayton, Ph.D.
Department of Medical Informatics
Intermountain Health Care
University of Utah
Salt Lake City Utah, USA

Sherry Dodson, M.L.S.
Health Sciences Libraries
Health Sciences Center-35-7155
University of Washington
Seattle, Washington, USA

James S. Fine, M.D.
Department of Laboratory Medicine
University of Washington
Seattle, Washingoton, USA

Teresa Spellman Gamble, M.P.A.
University of Washington Physicians
Network
Seattle, Washington, USA

Cezanne Garcia, M.P.H., C.H.E.S.
University of Washington Medical
Center Patient & Family Education
Services
University of Washington
Seattle, Washington, USA

John P. Geyman, M.D.
Department of Family Medicine
University of Washington
Seattle, Washington, USA

James I. Hoath, Ph.D.
Academic Medical Center Information
Services
University of Washington
Seattle, Washington, USA

Peter J. House, M.H.A.
Department of Family Medicine
University of Washington
Seattle, Washington, USA

Jeffrey Hummel, M.D.
Department of Medicine
University of Washington
Seattle, Washington, USA

Terry Ann Jankowski, M.L.S.
Healthy Sciences Libraries
Health Sciences Center-35-7155
University of Washington
Seattle, Washington, USA

Debra S. Ketchell, M.L., H.S.L.
Health Sciences Libraries
University of Washington
Seattle, Washington, USA

David Masuda, M.D.
Department of Medical Education,
Division of Biomedical and Health
Informatics
University of Washington
Seattle, Washington, USA

Thomas H. Payne, M.D.
Department of Medicine
University of Washington
Seattle, Washington, USA

Cedric J. Priebe III, M.D.
Department of Pediatrics
University of Vermont
Burlington, Vermont, USA

Eric Rose, M.D.
Department of Family Medicine
University of Washington
Seattle, Washington, USA

Sarah Safranek, M.L.I.S.
Health Sciences Libraries
Health Sciences Center-35-7155
University of Washington
Seattle, Washington, USA

Leilani St. Anna, M.L.I.S.
Health Sciences Libraries
Health Sciences Center-35-7155
University of Washington
Seattle, Washington, USA

Brent K. Stewart, Ph.D.
Department of Radiology
University of Washington
Seattle, Washington, USA

Anthony J. Wilson, M.D.
Department of Radiology
University of Washington
Seattle, Washington, USA

Fredric M. Wolf, Ph.D.
Department of Medical Education
University of Washington
Seattle, Washington, USA

1
Overview of Primary Care Informatics

THOMAS E. NORRIS, M.D.

Scenario 1

Setting: A Primary Care Office Practice without Functional Informatics Systems

The middle-aged family physician (FP) entered the exam room to see Alicia Jones, a 47-year-old female patient. He had provided care for Ms. Jones intermittently for years, so he was not too disturbed when Ms. Jones's chart could not be located (a situation that occurred several times each day in his practice). Her presenting complaint concerned a cough that produced blood. The history indicated that, within the 2 days prior to the visit, she had a morning cough that produced "several drops" of blood each day. The patient was a nonsmoker. After a physical examination of the lungs that was unremarkable, Ms. Jones was sent to the imaging center for a chest X ray. A short while later, the radiologist called the FP stating, "It looks like widespread lung metastases from the breast cancer we found on the mammogram 2 years ago. We will send the patient back up to your office so that you can talk with her about it."

The FP was shocked—he had never received the result of the mammogram, and he had not seen the patient in 2 years. The patient had never been told, by either the radiologist or the FP, about the positive screening mammogram, and she had received no treatment. Now, at the current visit, it appeared that metastatic disease was present. Ms. Jones returned from radiology to the primary care office. As her physician explained the situation, her demeanor changed from one of disbelief to one of extreme anger. After screaming at the physician, she stormed out of the office.

Ms. Jones expired, at age 48, from metastatic breast cancer (to lung, liver, and brain) several months later. Her family has filed a malpractice suit for delay in diagnosis of cancer against both the family physician and the radiologist, after the authorities denied attempts to have the physicians arrested on a criminal charge of murder.

Scenario 2

Setting: A Primary Care Office Practice with Functional Informatics

The middle-aged family physician entered the exam room and sat down with Ms. Andrea Smith, her 47-year-old female patient. Using the networked personal computer in the exam room, she opened the patient's electronic medical record (EMR) (Chapter 2, Electronic Medical Record). A quick review of the electronic problem list reminded the physician that the patient was being treated for breast cancer. The physician also noted that she had received in her "electronic in-basket" several important pieces of clinical data on the patient from other electronic sources (Chapter 3, Importing Data from Other Programs and Databases: HL7 Interfaces). Using the mouse to click on the "In-box" icon, she noted that some of the data were from her hospital laboratory. Another click on the lab icon revealed that the patient had a normal complete blood count (CBC), electrolytes, and creatinine—tests that had been run because the patient was receiving chemotherapy for breast cancer (Chapter 4, Importing Laboratory Data). The in-box also indicated that an imaging study had been completed and that the results had been returned to the chart. A click on the "Imaging" icon revealed a chest X-ray interpreted to be normal. A click on the "View film" icon caused the digital image of the film to appear on the exam room monitor, where the physician could review it and share it with the patient (Chapter 5: Importing Images).

In the ensuing discussion, due to upcoming international travel, the patient asked if she should get a hepatitis A immunization. She was concerned that, since she was immunosuppressed by her chemotherapy, the vaccine might be contraindicated. Since Ms. Smith was planning a vacation trip to Central America, her daughter had suggested that she might need to exercise special caution concerning communicable diseases that were found there. After checking two evidence-based medicine (EBM) Web sites and the Communicable Disease Center site on travel medicine, the FP felt that she could safely recommend the immunization (Chapter 6, Evidence-Based Medicine) and that it might provide useful protection in the countries that the patient planned to visit.

The patient also asked her physician to prescribe medication to prevent "traveler's diarrhea" on her trip. As the provider entered the prescription into the electronic order-writing tool in the EMR, a warning appeared, notifying her that the drug she had prescribed might be incompatible with one of Ms. Smith's chemotherapeutic agents (Chapter 7, Clinical Decision Support).

At the end of the visit, Ms. Smith asked if she should continue with the same oncologist, using the same medicines, or if she should consider switching to a new protocol she had heard about on a television talk show (and subsequently investigated by "surfing" the Web). Uncertain about the new protocol, the physician agreed to do some checking through the Web site of her local health sciences library and to e-mail the results to Ms. Smith—along with the newest patient information on her stage of breast cancer (Chapter 8, Knowledge Resources, and Chapter 9, Patient Education Resources and Instruction).

Just as she was leaving, the patient asked if the physician trusted the confidentiality of e-mailing personal information to her, and the physician briefly offered her opinions (Chapter 11, Privacy and Security of Patient Information).

Completing the visit, the physician said good-bye and went to the nurses' workstation outside the exam room, where she quickly approved several prescription refills, left responses to several telephone calls, and reviewed her schedule for the rest of the afternoon (Chapter 10, Workflow Automation with Electronic Medical Records).

While at the nurses' station, the physician closed out the breast cancer patient's chart, adding a CPT (Current Procedural Terminology) Code and an ICD-9 (International Classification of Disease) Code to the chart. At the end of the week, all the billings would be automatically transmitted to the appropriate insurance companies (Chapter 12: Electronic Billing for the Primary Care Physician).

At the end of the workday, the physician used the communications systems built into her clinical information system to answer and document a number of phone calls and e-mail messages from patients and colleagues (Chapter 14, Telecommunications in Primary Care).

Finally, before leaving the office at the end of the day, she used the information system to structure a query aimed at answering the question that had nagged her since her early-afternoon encounter with the 42-year-old breast cancer patient— How many cases of breast cancer had she seen in her practice, and were there any commonalties in the histories or demographic profiles of the patients? (Chapter 13, Reporting and Analysis).

Medical Informatics: What Is It and Why Should We Care?

Although many definitions have been used, medical informatics can be conveniently thought of as the discipline that concerns the management of medical information and the conversion of the information into useful knowledge. As the amount of information available to healthcare providers increases, medicine depends increasingly on efficient and comprehensive information management. No longer is it possible for physicians to maintain in their heads a storehouse of all of the basic and clinical knowledge they have gained, as well as pertinent historical information about the patient they are currently seeing. Instead of serving as walking storehouses of data, physicians must become integrators of information, with the skills to turn the information into knowledge on which rational actions can be based (Figure 1.1).

We live in an era in which the magnitude of new basic and clinical scientific data, as well as the specific information available about any single patient, is far too vast to depend on human memory for quick and efficient access. We have also passed the point at which the use of printed information in books, journals, or patient charts provides an adequate "auxiliary memory." The most rational approach to the situation is integrated electronic access using "smart tools" to multiple sources of data that are being continuously updated. Human primary care providers must shift from the role of acquirers and retainers of information

DATA ⇨ INFORMATION ⇨ KNOWLEDGE

FIGURE 1.1. Flow of data to knowledge.

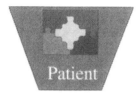

FIGURE 1.2. The patient is the focal point of care.

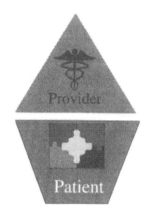

FIGURE 1.3. A good interpersonal relationship between the health care provider and the patient is an essential component of primary care.

to the role of integrators and manipulators of information—as well as *creators of knowledge.*

How Should the Primary Care Provider View Medical Informatics?

To understand the role of informatics in primary care, it is useful to return to basic concepts. The centerpiece of primary care is and always has been the patient (Figure 1.2) and the interpersonal relationship between a patient and a healthcare provider (Figure 1.3).

Historically, as the amount of information collected in the relationship between the patient and the primary care provider increased, the information was compiled and stored. At first, it resided in the memories of the provider and patient. When writing was developed, ancient physicians began to record information about patients. Classically, this information included the patient's perception of the disease process (history), as well as data based on the physical examination and other data developed by the provider. Beginning in the 1960s and 1970s, early medical informaticists began to organize this "chart" data in a logical way around problem lists in problem-oriented medical records (POMRs), with entries structured as "SOAP" (subjective, objective, assessment, plan) notes. This information formed the medical record. The Institute of Medicine (IOM) defines a patient record as follows:

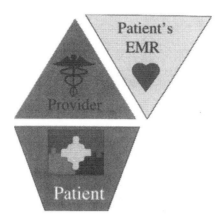

FIGURE 1.4. The electronic medical record (EMR) provides storage of and easy access to a lifetime of health data for patients.

> the repository of information about a single patient. Healthcare professionals gener-
> ate this information as a direct result of interaction with a patient or with individu-
> als who have personal knowledge of the patient (or with both). Traditionally patient
> records have been paper and have been used to store patient data.

As progress is being made with electronic hardware and software, the paper chart is evolving into an electronic medical record (EMR—also called computerized patient record, or CPR). A conceptual view is illustrated in Figure 1.4.

In 1991, the IOM's Computer-based Patient Record Institute (CPRI) made the following suggestion:[1]

> The committee recommends that healthcare professionals and organizations adopt
> the computer-based patient record (EMR or CPR) as the standard for medical and all
> other records related to healthcare.

The IOM and CPRI provide the following definition:[1]

> A Computerized Patient Record (CPR), also referred to as an Electronic Medical
> Record (EMR), is an electronic patient record that resides in a system specifically
> designed to support users by providing accessibility to complete and accurate data,
> alerts, reminders, clinical decision support systems, links to medical knowledge, and
> other aids.

CPRI continues:

> A Computerized Patient Record is electronically stored information about an indi-
> vidual's lifetime health status and healthcare.

Clearly a number of things must be included in the EMR, in addition to the paper chart emulation, for an EMR to meet the CPRI definition. These additional functions are represented graphically in Figure 1.5.

The last step in grasping the idea of primary care informatics as a system of handling medical data, with the EMR as its heart, is the need to incorporate the current trend toward more patient ownership of healthcare. A clear trend in the past

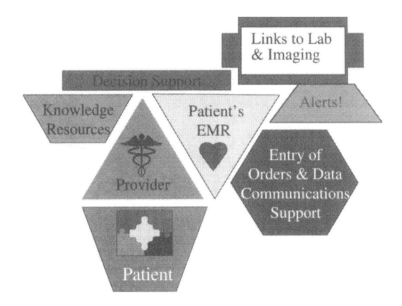

FIGURE 1.5. These additional elements make use of the electronic medical record (EMR) an asset.

few decades has been away from the traditional paternalistic model that had previously characterized healthcare toward a new paradigm in which patients are encouraged to take ownership of their health and of any disease processes that exist. Patient ownership requires both a new type of relationship between the patient and the physician and patient involvement in the acquisition, research, and compilation of their health data into the EMR. This concept is illustrated in Figure 1.6.

Why Should Primary Care Providers Use Informatics and EMRs?

Medicine has been somewhat suspicious of the ideas encompassed in medical informatics, and it has been slow to adopt EMRs. In general, medicine has applied the old aphorism "If it ain't broke, don't fix it." In the early 1990s CPRI suggested that, by the end of the decade, all medical records should be stored in electronic formats. As this chapter is being written early in 2001, this change has not happened. Yet almost 10% of primary care records are being recorded and compiled electronically, and the proportion of primary care providers using EMRs is increasing daily.

Several very strong forces are moving us toward better information management and electronic medical records.[2,3] First and perhaps most important is the desire to offer our patients the highest-quality healthcare possible. This goal cannot be accomplished when the provider is unable to find the records during an encounter with a patient, or is unable to read the poor handwriting in the records, or

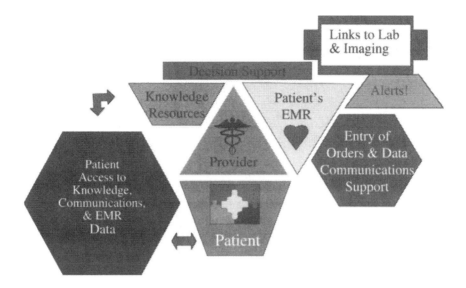

FIGURE 1.6. A good physician-patient relationship is essential to facilitating the accuracy and completeness of the EMR.

finds that the records are incomplete because lab and imaging results have not been filed. While all these problems can be addressed in the paper chart, they are more easily solved in the EMR. Additionally the EMR can enhance quality by including knowledge resources, such as practice guidelines, that can assist the provider in minimizing variation between his practice and "optimal" practices.[4]

In late 1998, the IOM published a widely heralded study on errors in medicine and error prevention. In reviewing their recommendations, it is clear that some of the most frequent errors could be avoided with the electronic order entry and decision support tools that are included in full-function EMRs. For example, if all prescriptions were legible and if all medication orders were automatically checked against a patient's allergies and for adverse interactions with the other drugs the patient is taking, then a large proportion of the mistakes that are currently being made could easily be avoided.[5]

Another reason to move toward medical informatics and electronic medical records is to improve service to patients and to improve their satisfaction with their care. If the patient's records cannot be found for a high percentage of visits, if imaging and laboratory results are frequently unfiled or filed in the wrong place (or in the wrong chart), and if the chart can be accessed by only one person in one place at one time, then patients will frequently receive poor service that will not promote their satisfaction with their healthcare. Imagine, for a moment, what it would be like if the airlines still kept all ticket information on handwritten slips of paper that are available only in one place at one time—if they can be read. Modern air travel would not be possible.

If you ask most employers (health care purchasers) to identify the single biggest problem in healthcare today, they will point to cost. One of the strongest arguments for adoption of good medical informatics practices coupled with the use of EMRs is controlling costs. Although adoption of EMRs and transition from paper records is expensive, these systems could help to stabilize and perhaps decrease the costs of care. Avoiding rework, the ordering of duplicate tests, inappropriate diagnostic and therapeutic measures, and errors would allow us to realize significant cost savings. Informatics and EMRs offer the promise of moving toward these goals. Another possible area of cost saving that these systems offer is a decrease in "transaction costs." Linking clinical documentation information to the bill for the service and then transmitting the bill electronically would reasonably be expected to decrease the business transaction cost of a healthcare encounter.

Why Is Now a Good Time to Move Forward with Informatics and EMRs?

Significant progress has been made in both practical applications of informatics theories and in so-called "base technologies." In 2000, the Robert Wood Johnson Foundation and the Institute for the Future presented a major report, *Health and Healthcare 2010: The Forecast, the Challenge.*[6] In the report they suggested that progress in the area of health care information management will depend on developments in base technologies. Let us examine the importance and status of each item in their list of base technologies:

- *Microprocessors*   Microprocessors serve as the core or "brain" of computers. Moore's law suggests that they will double in power every 1 to 2 years, and recent experience suggests that costs will continue to fall. Electronic medical information management, with user-friendly "intuitive" functionality, will depend on continued increases in computing power.
- *Data storage*   The development of low-cost lasers, compact discs, and optical storage systems has dramatically lowered the cost of data storage (memory) in recent years. Cheap data storage, coupled with the capacity to easily search, process, analyze, and retrieve the data, is a critical technology for progress in medical information management.
- *Software tools*   Stated simply, software is the set of instructions that allows a computer to accomplish a task. Over the past several decades progress has been made in the area of creating better, easier-to-use software and in the area of developing tools that allow people without programming training to build their own software. A major reason for the delay in the widespread adoption of EMRs, as well as the expense, is the borderline adequacy of the software that had been available. As improvements occur in these fields, this once formidable barrier is continually eroding.
- *Networking and data compression*   A significant trend in computer system design over the past 20 years has been a trend away from large, free-standing "mainframe" computers toward integrated networks of smaller computers and

personal computers (PCs). This new approach is called a "client-server" model. Development of networks has depended on the creation of new types of networking software, algorithms and protocols for compression of data, allowing it to be transmitted from one computer to another, and broad bandwidth transmission capabilities that allow huge files to be easily shared by multiple sites. Practical implementation of EMRs will depend heavily on this technology.

- *Information appliances*   While the computer is the most common information appliance, we will increasingly see the functions of computers appear in other equipment. Among current examples are electrocardiogram machines that provide interpretations of the tracings and home blood glucose monitors that "remember" a patient's blood sugar readings for the past month or more. These systems, especially when they are linked by interfaces to the EMR, will allow further progress in medical informatics.

- *Intelligent agents*   Intelligent agents are software programs that find and retrieve information for a user, based on the user's instructions to the agent. The most recognizable current examples include the National Library of Medicine's MedLine and PubMed systems, as well as the ubiquitous search engines used to locate information on the World Wide Web. While Medline searches can access voluminous original research literature on a given subject, many providers would find search engines that access filtered, peer-reviewed secondary data much more useful. Some progress is being made in the development of specialized search engines.[7] If the data stored in EMRs is going to be useful in either individual- or population-based medicine, further development of "intelligent agents" will be critically important.

- *Security and encryption*   Another area of great concern to both physicians and patients that must be addressed prior to widespread EMR use is data security and encryption. Fortunately, the financial and banking industries have experience in this field. The soon-to-be-implemented federal HIPAA (Health Insurance Portability and Accountability Act) legislation will require and promote progress in the healthcare arena.

- *Internet and World Wide Web*   These systems provide a common format for "viewing, exchanging, and transacting information of all kinds that is transferrable among different computer systems."[1] While the long-term implications of the Internet for healthcare are not clear, patients are currently increasingly seeking health information from "e-sources." In 1999, 70 million Americans used the Internet to seek health information, and this number is growing rapidly.[8] Among the major changes that the Internet will impose on health care, patient access to information (perhaps including their own EMR) and patient capacity to communicate with their physicians through e-mail will undoubtedly be significant.

- *3-D computing*   To date, most of the healthcare applications of the capacity to visualize data in three dimensions on a computer screen have been in imaging, but it is quite possible that other developments will arise in management of huge quantities of data.

- *Databases* Significant effort is being expended in the development of new relational and object-oriented databases. Goals include creation of systems that store larger amounts of data and allow better search capabilities. Even though new databases may be incompatible with older systems, progress must be made to manage the vast quantities of healthcare data in an efficient, integrated fashion.
- *Sensors* One likely advance in the next 10 years will be an increase in the availability and a decrease in the cost of biomedical sensors that will allow monitoring of many physiological and metabolic functions. Furthermore, it may become possible to easily integrate these data into the EMR.
- *Expert systems* The term "expert system," often used interchangeably with the term "decision support system," is applied to software that suggests options and outcome probabilities, as well as supporting the user in making decisions of many types. One of the great hopes for medical informatics and EMR's is that these systems will be able to aid primary care providers in real time settings in patient care.

These base technologies have set the stage for significant progress in applying medical informatics (and the EMR) to an ever-increasing number of patients and clinical settings. In addition, potential future developments in many of these areas, as well as in areas not readily anticipated at this time, offer hope that there may be excellent solutions for problems in healthcare that currently seem insoluble.

Where Will Things Go from Here?

To quote the Robert Wood Johnson report, "The direction is clear, the pace uncertain."[6] The next few steps, at least, seem fairly obvious. We need expanded knowledge among physicians and other healthcare providers about medical informatics. We also need to actively move toward complete, widespread implementation of electronic medical records systems. The groundwork for these steps has been laid, and it is probably time to move forward.

Clearly other developments in software, hardware, and networking will occur—many very soon. Among those that are either here or on the horizon are much greater use of voice recognition transcription, patient access to their medical records via a password-protected Web site, and practical use of wireless and perhaps hand-held computing devices in networked systems available in both ambulatory and in-patient settings.

Instead of spending too much time and effort trying to anticipate future developments, we need to use the capabilities available to us now to a much fuller extent than we are currently doing. Movement in this direction could result in better, cheaper, more satisfying care for our patients.

References

1. Computer-based Patient Record Institute (CPRI) 1995. *Proceedings of the First Annual Nicholas E. Davies CPR Recognition Symposium.* Ed. E.B.Steen, Schaumburg, IL: CPRI.

2. Wager KA, Ornstein SM, Jenkins RG. Perceived value of computer-based patient records among clinician users. *MD Computing* 1997;14(5):334–340.
3. Sullivan F, Mitchell E. Has general practitioner computing made a difference to patient care? A systematic review ot published reports. *BMJ* 1995;311: 848–852.
4. Tierney WM, Overhage JM, Takesue BY, Harris LE, Murray MD, Vargo DL, McDonald CJ. Computerizing guidelines to improve care and patient outcomes: The example of heart failure. *JAMIA, TN* 1995;2:316–322.
5. Bhasale AL, Miller GC, Reid SE, Britt HO. Analysing potential harm in Australian general practice: An incident-monitoring study. *Medical Journal of Australia* 1998;169:73–76.
6. Institute for the Future. *Health and Health Care 2010: The Forecast, the Challenge.* San Francisco: Jossey-Bass 2000;109–122.
7. Ebell MH. Information at the point of care: Answering clinical questions. *J Am Board Fam Pract* 1999;12:225–235.
8. Kleinke JD. Release 0.0: Clinical information technology in the real world. *Health Aff* (Millwood) 1998;17(6):23–28.

2
Electronic Medical Record (EMR)

HAROLD I. GOLDBERG, M.D.

The Three Rs

When many primary care physicians hear the phrase "electronic medical record," what comes to mind is a jumble of text, numbers, and images flickering on a monitor in front of their eyes. The purpose of this chapter is to present an alternative approach to thinking about EMRs. The basics of elementary education have traditionally been summarized as the three *R's*—reading, 'riting and 'rithmetic. The basics of elementary EMR education analogously are three Rs—reposit, report, and research. By concentrating on what we want computers to do for physicians, much of the hardware and software jargon that often plagues discussions about clinical computing can be dispensed with. This is a good thing because computer technology is rapidly evolving. Regrettably, many of the technical concepts referred to in the ensuing chapters may well be obsolete by the time this book finds its way to most of its eventual readership. The functionalities alluded to, in contrast, will endure.

This chapter is organized simply. First, a general discussion of the three Rs defines EMR functions and introduces the range of related terminology that can be overheard whenever physicians who are informatics-technology (IT) professionals sit down to lunch together. I have chosen the word "introduce" quite consciously; entire chapters are later devoted to discussing in detail the content implied by the various terms. Second, I present a case history of how the ambulatory EMR system currently used at the University of Washington Academic Medical Centers (UWAMCs) slowly came into being over the course of a decade. It is a story worth telling because—although certainly not the optimal way to build or buy an EMR system—it illustrates how the three Rs were developed and serially put into production. Finally, any discussions of EMRs should mention at least a few of the practical considerations facing those interested in purchasing systems here and now.

Reposit

Reposit refers to how the information that healthcare providers need is placed inside the computer and is stored for either immediate or later display. In practice, these data come from several sources. Information is often imported from other computers that specialize in capturing one particular type of data. Laboratory results come from the computer used to store test results. Results of X rays come from the computer into which transcriptions of interpretations dictated by radiologists are placed. In academic hospital settings, these computers are operated and maintained by separate departments. Thus, they are referred to as "departmental" computers. Because they generally were available long before the EMRs that sought to integrate their contents, they are also known as "legacy systems." Sometimes they are referred to as "source systems" containing "databases of record," implying responsibility for the accuracy of the information collected as it was originally created. This is opposed to "databases of reference," meaning the copies of information that support the integrative function of the EMR.

A commercial laboratory might find it necessary to send results to several clinic destinations in the same town. A hospital's billing computer might need to send information to several insurance companies to receive reimbursement for the complicated mix of services incurred during any single admission. This exchange of data is known as "interfacing." The rules employed so that exchanged data can be properly understood are called transmission "standards" and are represented by acronyms such as "HL7." Indeed, so much data may be flying around a large healthcare system at any time that a separate computer or "interface engine" is dedicated to accomplishing this exchange. If copies of data are sent the instant the original is generated, the interface is said to operate in "real time." Less important information can wait to be collected over a period of time before being transmitted over a "batch" interface.

Other information enters the EMR more directly. Physicians may type "free-text" notes from their keyboards or use "voice recognition" software to type for them. Notes of a repetitive nature can be partially prestored, requiring only the direct entry of items via a mouse-actuated "picklist." Such "templated" notation lends itself well to the more regimented types of data collection that physicians perform, such as a presurgical admission form or an operative report. Although diagnoses from billing data can be employed to generate problem lists, many physicians prefer to update or annotate problem lists with manually entered free text. Optical scanners can be employed to import simple images such as a handwritten note or an ophthalmologist's retinal doodle. More complex image "objects" can be captured directly. Many offices like to use digital cameras to include a snapshot of patients in their EMRs.

Once collected, all these kinds of information can be assembled into a single, large "relational" database. This means that laboratory data items in a "table" at one location of the storage medium can be related to, for example, demographic data items regarding the same patient in another table. These large databases have come to be known as "clinical data repositories (CDRs)" or "clinical data warehouses." Obviously, any EMR is only as good as the completeness and accuracy of all the information contained in its constituent CDR. Despite this fact, professionals ignominiously refer to all these databases and the maze of interfaces that support them as being the information system's "back end." Like the part of the horse that powers you to where you need to go—because it's invisible to the rider looking forward—CDRs get no respect.

Report

Reporting refers to the display of information for clinical use. This functionality is sometimes referred to as "results reporting" even though the types of data displayed go far beyond simple test results. The kinds of display devices usable are also numerous. Video monitors, flat-panel screens, or even the tiny liquid crystal displays on hand-helds and pagers are used. The look and feel of the information displayed mirrors that of the underlying operating system or "platform" that runs each device. EMR applications that run on Windows operating systems share the familiar look and feel of most Microsoft products. The display of EMRs that are browser-based are redolent of the average Web page. Newer "terminal-server" technologies that allow applications to be viewed remotely via a Web browser regardless of the underlying platform begin to blur such distinctions. Various EMR applications differ in the amount of data viewable on a given screen and the sophistication of its representation. A pager can successfully transmit a single critical lab value. More fully functional applications are able to display the entire panoply of text notes, numerical values, and images as individual items—as occurs in the traditional paper chart. Still more powerful EMRs are capable of processing the data at their disposal on the fly to create trended graphs or draw disparate data items relating to a chronic disease into a single coherent display.

Information other than that contained in the CDR can also be reported on. Some EMRs integrate "practice management" activities such as appointment scheduling, referrals, or billing to inform the clinical encounter and vice versa. In creating a note, for example, physicians can simultaneously generate a bill or schedule a subspecialty visit. Such abilities obviously have implications for who does what around the office, sometimes engendering thoroughgoing reexamination of practice workflow. Other EMRs incorporate external factual information known as "knowledge resources." These range from drug formularies to the contents of medical textbooks that can be checked at the point of service (POS)—that is, while the patient is being cared for. Web-based EMRs obviously extend the amount of factual information that can be displayed at the POS beyond data that can be stored locally.

Sometimes even clinical data are not stored locally inside Web-based EMRs. This is often the case with very large images. Like newspaper photographs composed of thousands of variously colored dots, a digitized EKG or X ray can be represented by millions of "binary digits (bits)" arrayed in two-dimensional "bitmaps." Rather than incur the expense of redundantly storing these "binary large objects" or "BLOBS" in both the databases of record and reference, a Web-based results reporter can be programmed to automatically "point" to the server storing the requested image remotely. The appropriate browser "plug-in" can then be called on to display the image as needed. The price paid for this efficiency is the encryption and other additional security measures required in transmitting clinical data over public networks.

Still, the promise of EMRs to provide the working physician with integrated displays of locally stored and remotely acquired clinical, factual, and management data of ever-increasing complexity is real. It's not surprising that front end bells and whistles grab so much attention.

Research

Research, in this context, does not refer specifically to experimentation. Instead, it means the intelligent analysis of data contained in the CDR for the purpose of providing clinical decision support. Such analyses can be performed in advance—that is, preprocessed. An example would be a "population monitor" that calculates each patient's status regarding recommended preventive maneuvers each evening. At any clinic visit, primary care providers can then be reminded of exactly who is due for mammograms or Pap smears, fecal occult blood testing or cholesterol determinations. Such analyses can also be performed in real time. Via "event monitors," physicians can be alerted whenever a patient is in the emergency room or has been admitted to the hospital. Intelligent order entry systems capable of avoiding drug-drug interactions can analogously operate in real time. Having the data stored in a single physical repository makes it possible to conduct these kinds of analyses with response times acceptable to the average provider.

Of course, such analyses can also be performed retrospectively. Coded feedback can be given comparing rates of glycemic control among groups of diabetic patients as a means of stimulating quality improvement interventions. This kind of activity is usually carried on by a software application known as a "query engine" or "report writer." The former often involves use of a "query language" unless commonly asked questions can be preprogrammed or "canned" in advance. The latter is a vendor-supplied product that can be applied to CDRs with minimal previous programming experience.

Without an ability to literally "re-search" the data stored in CDRs, little learning can take place from either individual patients or groups of patients over time. We cannot afford to squander the opportunity to use the vast cumulative evidence being generated every day in mainstream clinical settings to identify "best practices" and aid in the conduct of controlled trials that enhance "evidence-based" learning.

EMR Case History

The tripartite principle of reposit, report, and research has informed the development of the UW (University of Washington) clinical informatics capacity. The UWAMCs (University of Washington Academic Medical Center), located in Seattle, constitutes a unique resource in the Pacific Northwest of the United States. Their facilities include the only tertiary care hospital, level-one trauma center, and medical school available in the five contiguous "WWAMI" states of Washington, Wyoming, Alaska, Montana, and Idaho—an area equal to 27% of the United States landmass. Consistent with this regional mission, the construction of a large relational repository known as the Medical Information Networked Database (MIND) was undertaken in 1989. Its goal was to make both clinical and reference information available in real time to the primary and secondary care providers in the UW's far-flung referral base.

Originally, MIND employed interfaces with legacy registration, billing, pharmacy, laboratory, radiology, pathology, and transcription computing systems to generate text patient records that were viewable on the AMCs' local area network. In late 1995, however, clinical informaticists began to collaboratively design a graphical front end to the MIND repository using hypertext markup language (HTML), the authoring language used to create documents on the Web. This made MIND's contents accessible over the Internet using standard browsers such as Netscape Navigator or Microsoft's Internet Explorer. Security for this information tool, christened "MINDscape," was provided by secure socket layer (SSL) technology (a protocol developed by Netscape for encrypting communications) and a custom database application that authenticated users, managed passwords, and logged all accesses to the system. Faculty and residents also signed written confidentiality agreements and patients were given the opportunity to ask that their computerized records be accessible only in case of medical emergency. MIND presently stores the records of 612,000 patients in over 500 tables and 624,000,000 rows comprising a total of 115 gigabytes of data. A full-scale production system, each month 4000 users generate over 1.5 million MINDscape Web page "hits."

Independently, UW customer service liaisons had been working with two specialty practices across Puget Sound just west of Seattle and a large multispecialty clinic across the Cascade Mountains to the east. Staff had expressed increasing frustration over the continued inability to obtain copies of procedure notes and discharge summaries in advance of seeing patients who had returned home for follow-up care. In response, physicians at these three clinics became the first community providers given access to MINDscape in the spring of 1997, enabling them to remotely view the records of their identified patients under the pilot program "U-link." Dictated procedure notes, for example, could now be read on line as they were transcribed, often weeks before the receipt of hard copies through the mails. To date, 480 referring physicians have been enrolled in the pilot. With the support of conveniently integrated reference materials—such as PubMed, the National Library of Medicine's Web-based literature citation and retrieval system, and the UW-developed Federated Drug Reference—they have followed the care of 16,000 patients hospitalized in Seattle. Some have done so from as far away as Ketchikan, Alaska—a distance of 667 miles.[1]

Over the last two decades, numerous trials have confirmed the usefulness of computerized reminders in improving provider ordering behavior.[2] Applied most often to preventive maneuvers, point-of-service prompts had also been employed in chronic disease care. Developers of the MIND repository wanted the first decision support application written against this CDR to be of clear benefit. Accordingly, development of CROS (the Clinical Reminder and Outcome System) was

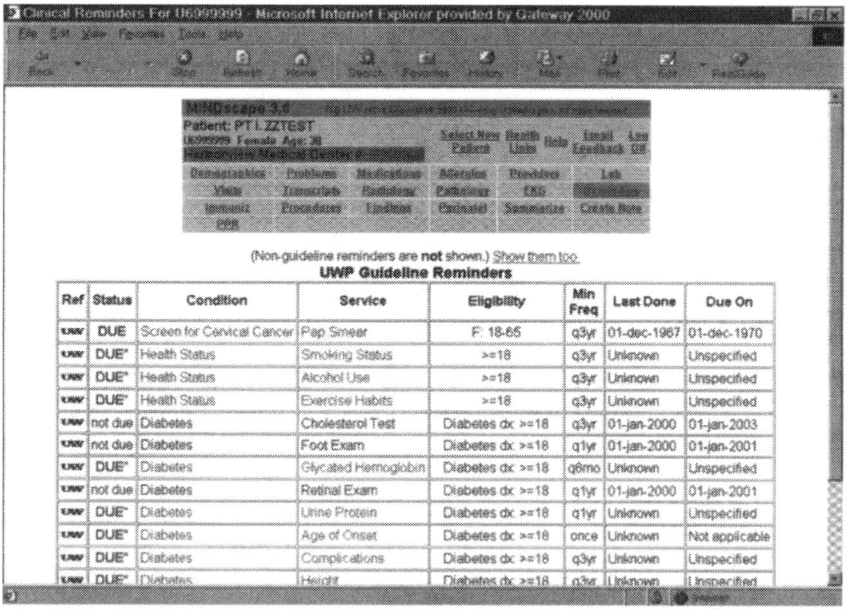

FIGURE 2.1. CROS reminders for the MINDscape test patient.

begun in 1995. A print screen of the reminders folder for the MINDscape "test patient" used for demonstrations is shown in Figure 2.1.

Over time, the reminder set has grown to include all the preventive maneuvers included in the Health Plan Employer Data and Information Set (*HEDIS*) performance measures required for accreditation of managed-care plans. Process measures for hypertension and diabetes, the first internal chronic disease guidelines written by University of Washington physician task forces have also been added. A unique feature of CROS is that it additionally prompts for collection of related physiologic outcomes such as blood pressure and glycated hemoglobin measurements, as well as measures of functional outcome and health status such as the SF-12. This expanded CROS reminder software was alpha-tested at the UW Family Medicine Center (FMC) as part of a 2-month implementation trial in late 1996. The FMC provides care to 7700 patients in a satellite facility a mile west of the medical school campus. Results included a mean relative increase in indicated ordering of 70%, including an increase of over 150% in mammography utilization.[3] Based on the success of this trial, the CROS software was successfully deployed at all 12 major UWAMC primary care clinics.

Two more recent enhancements to MINDscape have been the ability to directly enter data into the MIND repository over the Internet and the addition of a Web-based query engine that employs the standardized structured query language (SQL) to facilitate the routine analysis of stored information. Figure 2.2 displays the screen employed by faculty providers at an affiliated nursing home to enter

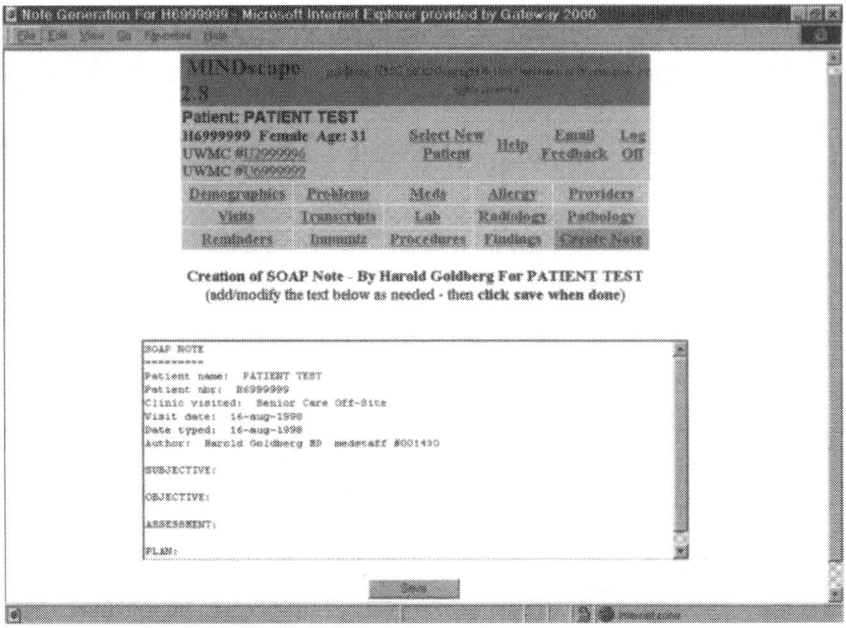

FIGURE 2.2. MINDscape note entry screen.

progress notes. By using the query engine—known as the MIND Access Project (MAP)—MIND contents are now available in a number of different forms. Raw data can be downloaded as Excel or ASCII text files from the individual tables where they are stored. This information can then be easily imported into local PC applications such as Access or SPSS for further manipulation and reporting. As an example, Figures 2.3 and 2.4 display early MAP screens that were used for documenting and downloading laboratory tests and results. The multiviews feature prejoins related information across several individual tables to facilitate the downloading process. Thus, data on the charges incurred by patient encounters can be abstracted in a single operation.

For end users unable to analyze raw data, MAP also provides a growing list of preprogrammed custom queries that can create commonly requested reports with a few mouse clicks. For example, Figure 2.5 shows the screen that can be used to create reports at either the clinic or the provider level regarding institutional guidelines for preventive and chronic disease care. Figure 2.6 shows clinic-level compliance with diabetes process measures at the FMC. Figure 2.7 shows a query concerning mammography compliance rates among the physicians practicing at the Adult Medicine Clinic located at Harborview Medical Center (HMC), the former county hospital now operated by the UW as a regional trauma center. Clicking on the coded hyperlinks in the left-hand column generates a canned query that lists patients currently not in compliance and contact information. Depending on complexity and the time of day when they are submitted, MAP queries generally

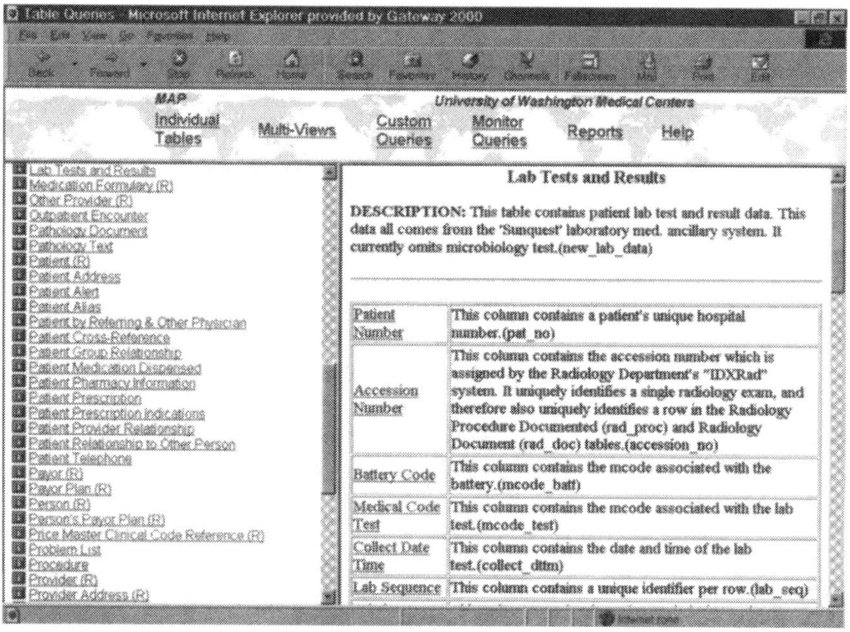

FIGURE 2.3. Description of data stored in MIND's "Lab Tests and Results" table.

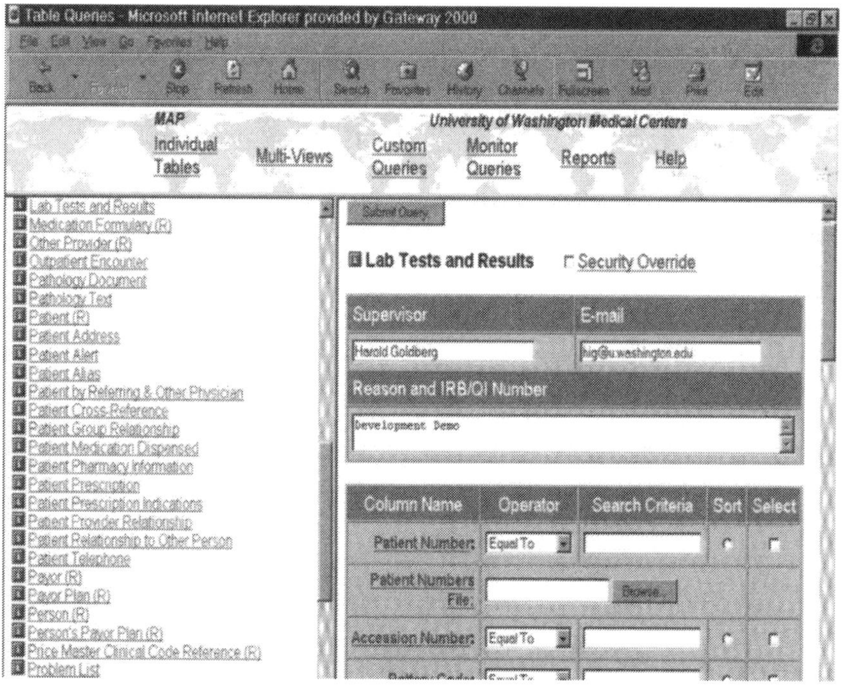

FIGURE 2.4. Selection of data stored for downloading.

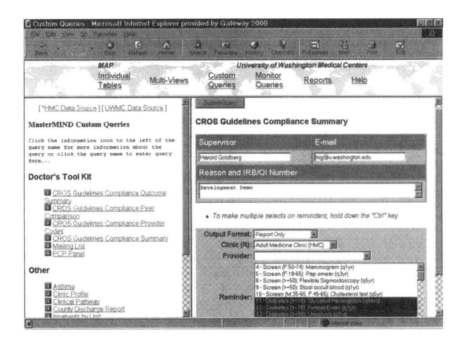

FIGURE 2.5. Generating a MAP report on compliance with selected diabetes items.

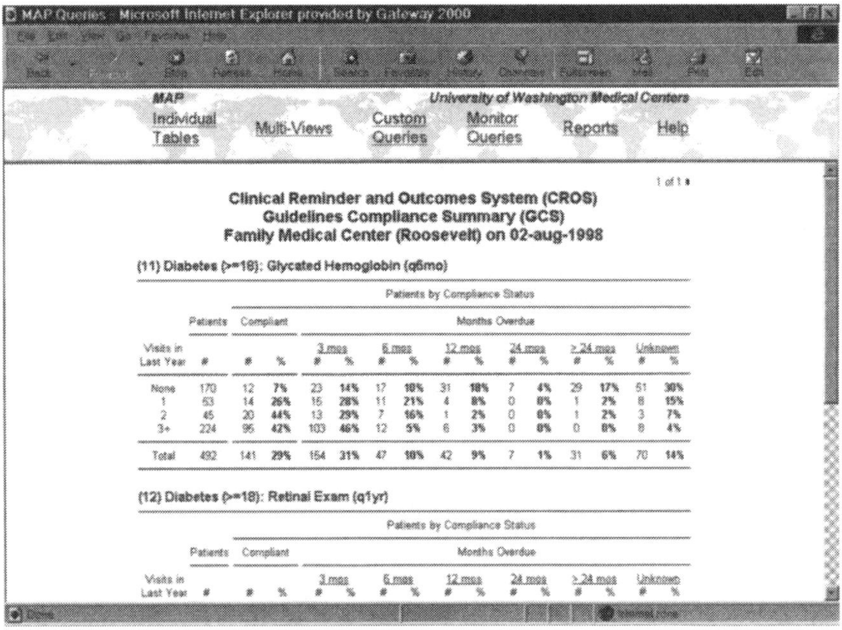

FIGURE 2.6. MAP diabetes compliance report at the clinic level.

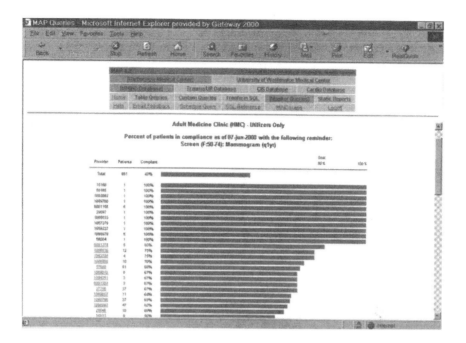

FIGURE 2.7. MAP mammography compliance report at the provider level.

take between 2 and 20 minutes to run. E-mail is automatically sent to inform the user when output is ready for viewing or downloading. Additionally, availability of MIND data has also allowed controlled trials to be conducted without supplementary chart abstraction.[3-5]

Purchasing Considerations

It is not this book's intention to instruct primary care physicians on how to purchase an EMR. We do, however, hope that those who make it through all the chapters will be in a better position to make an informed purchase. On the way to making the decision, additional resources might be consulted—especially those available on the Web itself. Industry nonprofit organizations, such as the Computer-based Patient Record Institute (CPRI), make a number of documents detailing the content and function of the platonic EMR available on their Web sites (www.cpri.org). A number of medical societies offer primers on selecting the proper system and approaching prospective vendors. A good example can be found at the site maintained by the American Academy of Family Practice's computerization clearinghouse (www.aafp.org/fpnet). Much can also be learned from visiting individual vendor sites. A list of 250 vendor links is available at the American Medical Informatics Association site (www.amia.org).

Four helpful hints are generally agreed to.

1. Define your actual needs carefully before approaching the marketplace. Even consider preparing a formal request for proposals listing what is desired.
2. Talk to your peers about their vendor experiences, what EMRs they've purchased and why. Take the time to make site visits after you narrow your search to one or two systems, asking pointed questions about negatives as well as positives. Do not buy based on a demonstration alone and beware of "vaporware" systems or modules that are not actually in production.
3. Fully understand and be prepared to negotiate all the costs involved. There is much more to be considered than just the initial licensing fee—and whether the fee is based on the number of staff who will be using the EMR and/or the volume of use. Learn about yearly maintenance fees and how charges for software updates, interfaces, and even training are handled. Be clear on who owns the data and any costs incurred in accessing and analyzing them.

   For all the benefits it will bring, implementing an office EMR system is a little bit like an extensive home remodel. It will probably cost twice as much and take twice as long as you originally expected. If you are comfortable with that, the experience can be a rewarding one. If the initial capital required appears daunting, investigate application service provider models where the EMR hardware and software is owned by the vendor who operates them for you—usually for a small per-patient per-year fee. In essence, youll be a renting an EMR instead of owning one.
4. Have a good lawyer familiar with information technology review any contract. Given that initial hardware and software costs for even a small group of practitioners are generally measurable in the hundreds of thousands of dollars, even honest negotiating mistakes can be expensive.

Conclusion

To be successful, EMR systems must collect, display, and analyze data—that is, reposit, report, and research. They are beginning to change how primary care is practiced, improve its quality, and enlarge its evidence base. As more clinics become computerized, these trends will surely accelerate.[6] As patients as well as providers begin to use this powerful tool at home over the Internet, we can only expect change to accelerate even faster.

References

1. Goldberg HI, Tarczy-Hornoch P, Stephens K, Larson EB, LoGerfo JP. Internet access to patients' records. *Lancet* 1998:351(9118):1811.
2. Shea S, DuMouchel W, Bahamonde L. A meta-analysis of 16 randomized controlled trials to evaluate computer-based clinical reminder systems for preventive care in the ambulatory setting. *J Am Med Inform Assoc* 1996;3:399–409.
3. Goldberg HI, Neighbor WE, Cheadle AD, Ramsey SD, Gore E, Diehr P. A controlled time-series trial of clinical reminders: Using computerized firm systems

to make quality-improvement research a routine part of mainstream practice. *Health Serv Res* 2000;34:1519–1534.

4. Goldberg HI, Wagner EH, Fihn SF, Martin DP, Horowitz CR, Christensen DB, Cheadle AD, Diehr P, Simon G. A randomized controlled trial of CQI teams and academic detailing: Can they alter compliance with guidelines? *Jt Comm J Qual Improv* 1998;24:130–142.

5. Taylor VM, Thompson B, Lessler D, Yasui Y, Montano D, Johnson KM, Mahloch J, Mullen M, Li S, Bassett G, Goldberg HI. A clinic-based mammography intervention targeting inner city women. *J Gen Intern Med* 1999;14: 104–111.

6. Goldberg HI, Horowitz CR. Musings on using evidence to guide CQI efforts toward success: The computerized firm system as primary care microunit. *Jt Comm J Qual Improv* 1999;25:529–538.

3
Importing Data from Other Programs and Databases: HL7 Interfaces

James I. Hoath, Ph.D.

Scenario

The timely and accurate acquisition of information (data) from multiple sources is important to the good care of a patient. As an example, consider a pediatrician who is evaluating a 6-year-old girl with short stature who has just moved into town. The first piece of information to acquire is the girl's growth chart from her previous caregiver. The next pieces of information to acquire are any laboratory values from any previous short stature workup—these values may be in the paper chart from the previous caregiver or they may reside on one or more centralized lab computers. Armed with this information the pediatrician can initiate the next steps in the workup, which may include some standard tests run at the local hospital, some much less common endocrine tests that are sent out to a national lab, and radiographic studies including potentially plain radiographs for bone age and, if indicated, an MRI of the hypothalamic-pituitary region. The more seamlessly the pediatrician is able to access the results of this diagnostic workup, the more efficiently care can be delivered—avoiding, for example, repeating tests when results are unavailable and evidence of a specimen having been sent is unavailable. In the paper world, transport, importation, and integration of this information takes place via fax, mail, manual collation of paper, and filing of paper into the paper record. The analogues in the electronic world are outlined in this chapter.

Need for Interfaces and Standards

All systems are made stronger, larger, or more successful as the flow of the substances that make them up are transported more effectively among the constituent parts. Just as a system of political states thrives when its transportation and communications paths are improved, or a living body thrives as its arteries and veins successfully exchange oxygen and wastes, so does an information system grow in power and effectiveness as its component parts exchange information. Healthcare information systems are no exception to this maxim, but they have historically lagged behind other industries in heeding its call.

The more the members of a multipart information system share information, the more able they are to meet the needs of the user community. This increases the dependency of one member on another, but it greatly strengthens the overall system. A radiology information system (RIS), for instance, can handle complex texts and images, but it can find itself at the mercy of fallible human data entry to tie this information to the right patient. A typo in the medical record number (MRN) can lead to results tied to the wrong patient and serious medical errors, whereas linking the RIS to a reliable, automated source of patient MRNs and other demographic information can prevent errors. Similarly, if the radiology results reside only in the radiology system, they are considerably less accessible to a referring provider who may or may not have access to the on-line RIS or to a phone interface to the RIS. Thus linkages from specialized information systems (e.g., RIS) to more general information systems (e.g., electronic medical records;— see Chapter 2) are also important.

Few would contest the idea that regular and reliable exchanges of data among the members of a set of healthcare systems would increase the utility of the individual systems and the value of the whole. The form and structure of the exchanges are not so easy to agree on. This chapter examines the history and architecture of one such set of forms and structures, which has evolved to become the primary formal standard for exchanges of data in the healthcare industry—HL7. We begin by reviewing the initial motivations for the standard, its goals, and its basic scope. We trace the highlights of its decade-long history, then turn to focus on its current state and achievements. A review of HL7's underlying methodology leads us to its goals for the future. We end with a description of its organizational structure and position in the broader context of other healthcare standards bodies. An important point to bear in mind is that though HL7 is a widely adopted standard in and of itself, it is not a guarantee that two systems that are both HL7 compliant can communicate and exchange data seamlessly.

HL7 Overview

As the other chapters point out, hospitals are seeing a dramatic rise in the use of computer-based information and diagnostic systems. What's more, the systems are usually a variety of independent, minicomputer- or microcomputer-based systems rather than a single large monolithic mainframe. The need to reduce both labor costs and medical errors resulting from redundant manual data entry has led to the search for increased communication among systems. This communication is analogous to human language: (a) basic meaning or semantics, (b) sentence structure or syntax, (c) the structure of individual "words" or elements in the "sentence," and (d) vocabulary. As with humans, there must be a shared understanding of all of these levels for real communication to occur. That is, in addition to the physical connection between systems, there must be a logical one. Providing this shared understanding is the goal of HL7. It does so by setting out a specific order or sequencing of data elements in a stream of data, definitions of how a data element is recognized—that is, where it starts and stops—and the format of individual items. Note that this specification and definition is not at the level of the physical hard-

TABLE 3.1 ISO/OSI information model protocol stack.

ISO/OSI Level
7. Application
6. Presentation
5. Session
4. Transport
3. Network
2. Data link
1. Physical

ware network or the data packets on them, but rather at the higher level of what the data actually means to a human. This explains the name of the standard, "Health Level Seven." "Seven" is the "Application Level," the highest and most abstract level of the *ISO/OSI* protocol stack (an international standards body specification) for communication of open systems (see Table 3.1). This is the level at which transported data is actually defined for use, the exchanges are triggered, message receipt is verified, and the message is timing set.

The goals for such an initiative are ambitious. The intent is to facilitate communication for all of the tasks that occur in a healthcare organization. The need for maximal standardization and interoperability on such a wide front of activity has to be balanced with a toleration for individual idiosyncrasy within the various systems and organizations. In such an undertaking as HL7, everyone can agree in theory that standardization is mandatory, but when representing individual organizations or data systems, these same people will hold out for "their" way. The standard must come to grips with this.

Another goal is to reduce the "spaghetti" inherent in the existence of many interfaces to and from many systems. Related to this is the goal to reduce the time and cost of an interface by leveraging the existence of a similar one. For instance, having written our interface of information outbound (going out) from the registration system to the radiology information system, we would ideally want to use the same outbound flow of data from the registration system for our new lab system, rather than starting from scratch.

Yet another goal is to increase the reliability of the data within the systems. This leads to the goal of a standard syntax than can be understood and used by all these systems. Finally, there is a need to facilitate the discussion or negotiation process between two groups preparing to implement an interface.

HL7 Evolution

The history of HL7 is not long, barely more than a decade. The standard and the organization that produces it grew out of a meeting held at the University of Pennsylvania in 1987 to establish some common ground in communication standards

between computers in healthcare. The participants faced an industry that had virtually no accepted standards. If only five systems wished to share data, essentially 20
($N*[N - 1]$) interfaces had to be built from scratch, each independent of the other,
each with its own standards, data formats, and vocabulary. That same year, the
group released an initial standard, Version 1.0, not much more than an initial draft.
This was quickly followed by a more comprehensive work, Version 2.0, the following year. This is essentially the version that developers have been using for the
last decade, although it has been updated by several hefty incremental additions:
Versions 2.1 in 1990, 2.2 in 1994, and the current Version 2.3 in 1996. Version 2.4
in 2001 is probably be the last in this series. In each of these 2.X versions the underlying syntax and control structures are the same, with entire new chapters appearing based on such healthcare functions as medical records, appointment scheduling, and automated lab devices. HL7 gained accreditation as an ANSI national
standard in 1994. The next version will be the long-heralded Version 3.0, representing a paradigm shift in the syntax. HL7 first began working on it in 1996. It dis-
cards the current syntax for one based on XML and is heavily dependent on structured vocabularies. We'll take a closer look at the activity in Version 3.0 later.

As HL7 evolved and progressed through the 1990s, its goals expanded. Since
the mid-1990s, increasing focus has been placed on the RIM, or reference information model, which serves as a formal data design and underlying guide for all
the data and information design done by HL7. This inevitably expands HL7's
scope into the area of overall data design for healthcare systems, rather than solely
for intersystem transport. This expansion in part has been necessitated by the need
to have not only a common vocabulary and messaging system but a common representation of the data across applications. HL7 development activity is now increasingly focused on shared and structured vocabularies so that cooperating systems share an unambiguous knowledge of the meaning of the data. A shared
vocabulary would address one of the limitations of HL7 today, which is that the
meaning of some data elements is not fully specified and is subject to differing interpretation by different vendors implementing HL7 interfaces. HL7 has taken on
defining the data for the functions of clinical decision support (CDS) systems. A
relatively new group has taken on data security. Another technical committee
(CCOW) is defining the specifications for how all applications open on a desktop
would exchange information about their current context, that is, who the user is
and which patient and type of data the application should be focused on. Yet another group is developing a model clinical document architecture (CDA) for the
exchange of a wide range of documents that lays the groundwork for a shared definition of the EMR (see Chapter 2). As HL7 goals have expanded, its traditional
pragmatism toward the concept of "plug-and-play" is gradually shifting. Plug-
and-play is the idea that two systems literally plug themselves into each other and
the interface of data immediately begins to work perfectly, out of the box. The
term "interoperability" has always been an HL7 watchword, capturing the intent
to maximize data sharing within practical limits but avoiding the self-defeating
holy grail of plug-and-play expectations. The issue is that the older HL7 specifications were ambiguous enough that rarely did two HL7 compliant systems communicate seamlessly; additional custom interface work was frequently needed

(within the HL7 constraints). The use of a common information model (the RIM) and promulgation of unambiguous shared vocabularies brings us several steps closer to that ideal.

In just 12 years HL7 has become an integral part of the systems development process for all major healthcare vendors and institutions. Few hospitals would now even consider buying or building a system without HL7 inputs and outputs. As HL7 has itself become an industry, a number of vendors have emerged with products that centralize and manage the traffic of data among the systems. These products are high-level data routers, but they have become known as interface engines. As interface traffic has proliferated within hospitals and the sophistication of the vendors' products has improved, most organizations have moved from internally developed interface engines to those of the vendors.

Despite HL7's embrace of vocabulary definition, information modeling, security standards, clinical decision support, and interapplication context synchrony, it is still primarily an organization and standard that manages the transport of data among systems, and there are limits to its scope. HL7 doesn't deal with the storage of data within a system, at any level, even though the RIM suggests a nudge in that direction. There is no requirement for a programming language. The lower six layers of the ISO stack ("network" through "presentation") are not specified, although as we'll see later some lower level protocols (LLPs) are offered as suggestions. A communicating system can have any internal architecture. Any one of the messaging types can be implemented without the others.

HL-7 Implementation Details: HL7 2.X Standards

We began by describing HL7 as akin to a human language. The structure of this language is laid out in the various chapters of the *HL7 Standard,* and there is generally an HL7 technical committee responsible for each chapter. The product of the technical committees is sometimes augmented by work from the SIGs, or special interest groups. It was the master patient index (MPI) SIG, for instance, that developed the MPI query and request messages for the patient administration chapter.

We examine the HL7 2.X standard (meaning any of the Version 2s) by focusing on selected individual chapters and the functions they describe. The intent is to illustrate via example the complexity of the HL7 standard, the areas where ambiguity is currently possible, and by extension, the challenge posed by the need to interface disparate systems. From the point of view of the primary care provider the important points are (a) compliance with HL7 is not a guarantee of plug-and-play, and (b) development of interfaces from ancillary systems (radiology, laboratory, and so on) to an electronic medical record system is a significant challenge.

Chapter 2: Control

This chapter defines the basic building blocks on which all the subsequent chapters and message types are based:

TABLE 3.2 Examples of ADT messages.

ADT message	
MSH	Message header (ADT)
EVN	Event type (A08)
PID	Patient-specific information and identifiers
NK1	Next-of-kin information
PV1	Patient visit information

- The form to be used in describing all messages, their purpose, their contents, and the interrelationships among them. This form is called an "abstract" message definition because it operates at the top, or seventh, or most abstract (application) level of the ISO/OSI model.
- The acknowledgment message, a special message that is used across all applications to acknowledge all the other (unsolicited update) messages.
- Message segments that are common to all messages.
- The HL7 encoding rules for representing the abstract information of a communication as a string of characters that make up the physical message.
- The programming procedures required to exchange messages using the HL7 specifications.
- Suggested relationships to the lower level protocols.

Trigger Events. Messages begin their life with a "trigger event," a real-world event that causes a message to be sent out. The trigger event is tied to a specific message type. HL7 takes considerable care in standardizing on the trigger events the message types, the messages' internal structure, and the encoding rules. Using our earlier example, the registration system responsible for tracking and sending patient information would be triggered by an "Update patient information" event to send out a message of message type ADT, trigger event "A08," to the radiology information system.

Messages. The message is the smallest meaningful entity that can be transferred from one system to another. Messages comprise segments, which themselves comprise fields. If we continue the analogy to human language, trigger events are real-world actions with meaning, messages are paragraphs, segments are sentences, and fields are words. The trigger event "Update patient information" creates an ADT message (paragraph) with a number of segments (sentences) in it, each concerning a particular type of data. The EVN segment describes the trigger event, the PID segment carries patient-specific data, the PV1 carries patient visit information, the NOK segment carries next-of-kin information, and so on. Some of these segments are required, others are optional, and some can repeat (Table 3.2).

Acknowledgment Messages. The acknowledgment message or ACK notifies the sender that the receiver actually got the message. Note that the underlying

TABLE 3.3 Abstract message syntax for an ADT/AO8 message "Update patient information."

ADT	ADT message
MSH	Message header
EVN	Event type
PID	Patient identification
[PD1]	Additional demographics
[{NK1}]	Next of kin/Associated parties
PV1	Patient visit
[PV2]	Patient visit—additional information
[{DB1}]	Disability information
[{OBX}]	Observation/Result
[{AL1}]	Allergy information
[{DG1}]	Diagnosis information
[DRG]	DRG information
[{PR1	Procedures
[{ROL}]	Role
}]	
[{GT1}]	Guarantor information
[	
{IN1	Insurance information
[IN2]	Insurance information—Additional information
[IN3]	Insurance information—Cert.
}	
]	
[ACC]	Accident information
[UB1]	Universal bill information
[UB2]	Universal bill 92 information

Square brackets indicate that a segment or group of segments is optional; curly braces indicate that segments may repeat.

communications-layer protocols are not deemed sufficient to guarantee delivery of the message. We must know that the receiving application processed the data successfully at its own seventh application level.

Segments, Fields, and Components. Segments are made up of a series of fields in a defined order, much as English sentences are series of words in a required order. A segment always begins with the three-letter code that denotes its function, such as PID for "patient information/demographics." The order of the field defines its semantic role. For instance, field 6 in the PID segment is always "Mother's maiden name." Fields themselves can be subdivided into smaller units called components.

Encoding Rules. These rules inform the specification of the characters to be used for separating segments from each other (the carriage return), as well as defaults for separating fields and repeating fields and components. This is also where a particular character set can be defined. The default is printable ASCII characters.

In Table 3.3 is the abstract message syntax for our ADT/A08 message "Update patient Information." Square brackets indicate that a segment or group of segments is optional; curly braces indicate that they may repeat.

TABLE 3.4 Examples of trigger events in patient administration.

Trigger event	Message
Admit a patient/Start a visit	A01
Transfer a patient	A02
Discharge a patient/End a visit	A03
Register a patient	A04
Preadmit a patient	A05
Change an outpatient to an inpatient	A06
Update patient information	A08
Swap patients	A17

Z messages and Z Segments. In addition to the message and segments defined by the HL7 chapters for general use, the abstract message syntax outlined in Table 3.3 can be used by individual developers to craft their own message types and segments. The naming convention used is to start the three-letter code with a Z. This ability to create custom message types and segments is one of the reasons the plug-and-play ideal is difficult to achieve. On the other hand it is a very powerful feature that permits developers to create custom messages that are tailored to a particular application.

Chapter 3: Patient Administration

This was the first application-specific chapter to be developed in any detail. This is hardly surprising, since it represents the applications that own the information most needed: who and where the patient is. The trigger events and transactions in this chapter are those known as registration and ADT (admit/discharge/transfer) events (Table 3.4). There are 50 other messages, triggered by such events as "Cancel leave of absence," "Cancel patient's return from leave of absence," "Change consulting doctor," "Cancel change of consulting Doctor," and so on.

Chapter 4: Order Entry

This chapter describes the structure of the messages used for ordering something from within one system and sending the order to the "filling" system. Unlike patient administration with its 60 message types for various trigger events, order entry has only three generic message types, with room for variation provided by the many segment definitions within the messages (Table 3.5). This gives us orders for observation and diagnostic studies in lab medicine, radiology, pathology,

TABLE 3.5 Examples of trigger events in order entry.

Trigger event	Message
General order message	ORM
General order response message (as a response to the ORM)	ORR
Query/response for an order's status	OSQ

TABLE 3.6 Examples of trigger events in financial management.

Trigger event	Message
Add a patient account	P01
Purge the patient's accounts	P02
Post financial detail transactions	P03
General bills and accounts receivable	P04
Update a patient account	P05
End a patient account	P06

TABLE 3.7 Examples of trigger events in observation reporting.

Trigger event	Message
Unsolicited request	ORU
Purge the patient's accounts	QRY

and diagnostic/therapeutic areas. It also handles pharmacy and dietary requests, as well as requests for immunizations.

Chapter 6: Financial Management

The messages for these six events handle the entry and manipulation of information on patient billing accounts, charges, payments, claims adjustments, insurance, and other related patient billing and accounts receivable information (Table 3.6).

Chapter 7: Observation Reporting

This chapter deals with exchanging structured patient-oriented clinical data among systems. Typical use would be to transmit observations and results of diagnostic studies from the producing system, such as a clinical laboratory system or an EKG or EMG system to the ordering system, such as an order entry or physician's office system. Like the order entry chapter (Chapter 4), there are few trigger events but a rich variety of segments within the messages (Table 3.7). These messages are often the second part of the ordering loop, after an order message. The observations can be sent from producing systems to archival medical record systems and other systems that were not part of the ordering loop, e.g., an office practice system of the referring physician for inpatient test results ordered by an inpatient surgeon. These same message structures are used to send waveform observations. Recent work provides mechanisms for registering clinical trials and methods for linking orders and results to clinical trials and for reporting adverse patient experiences with drugs and devices. There are an additional 15 trigger events that are used solely for messaging around clinical trials and product experiences.

TABLE 3.8 Examples of trigger events in information management.

Trigger event	Message
Original document notificaton	T01
Original document notification and content	T02
Document status change notification	T03
Document status change notification and content	T04
Document addendum notification	T05
Document addendum notification and content	T06
Document edit notification	T07
Document edit notification and content	T08
Document replacement notification	T09
Document replacement notification and content	T10
Document cancel notification	T11

Chapter 9: Medical Records/Information Management

While currently limited to the basic medical records functions listed in Table 3.8, this chapter should soon handle other medical record functions, including chart location and tracking, deficiency analysis, consents, and release of information.

Chapter 11: Patient Referrals

This chapter defines messages used in patient referral communications between mutually exclusive healthcare entities, such as from a community-based primary care clinic to a hospital-based specialty clinic. The 15 trigger events revolve around the information needed to automate this process. Much of the activity deals with the treatment that an insurance plan would authorize for a given patient.

Chapter 12: Patient Care

The messages in this chapter support the communication of problem-oriented records, including clinical problems, goals, and pathway information among systems.

Chapter 13: Clinical Laboratory Automation

Communication between automated devices, such as monitors, and a lab information system (LIS) is defined with 11 trigger events in this new chapter for Version 2.4.

Summary

HL7's Chapter 2, Control, provides the architecture for all HL7 messages, and the subsequent chapters provide a rich smorgasbord of functional, application-specific messages. The HL7 Working Group's intent is to continue developing as many new functional message types as possible. Where a particular type of message or segment may be lacking, the developer may construct a custom Z message or Z segment.

The success of HL7 in the United States and the rest of the world is due in large part to its methodology, both formal and informal. HL7 combines bullish, heads-down, "just do it" pragmatism (present from the beginning) with a growing reliance on a formal process and tools to derive content from formal information modeling. HL7 technical committees have rarely been reluctant to put out an imperfect standard. With "Perfection is the enemy of good" as their motto they have relied on getting the "correct" 80% of useful transactions out and in use as soon as possible, then turning around to perfect the remaining 20% over a longer period. While this practice led to some anomalous specification in the early years, it has ultimately resulted in a set of standards timely enough yet broad and comprehensive enough to warrant acceptance by the health care community.

Reference Information Model

All the Version 3.0 work and much of the work for Versions 2.3 and 2.4 has relied on a formal data model called the reference information model (RIM). This tool models and documents the data content and relationships of the objects in healthcare, for instance "patient" and "encounter." RIM is accompanied by a domain information model (DIM). The two are now the underlying semantic representation for all HL7 endeavor. Another formal tool in use since Version 2.3 is use cases. These are real-world scenarios that indicate and document how a message will be used by the people and systems it involves. HL7 working groups now follow a standard process in developing new message types, using use cases and basing the data on the RIM. This adherence to a comprehensive, static data model will likely move HL7 closer to developing parts of an electronic health record.

4
Importing Laboratory Data

James Fine, M.D., and David Chou, M.D.

Scenario 1

You have just completed a patient history and physical exam. You determine that the patient needs laboratory tests to rule out secondary hypertension. You pull out and fill out paper requisition forms for basic blood work. You send the patient to the laboratory phlebotomist servicing the practice with a requisition for a basic seven-test chemistry profile (CHEM7) and a complete blood count (CBC). The patient goes home with filled-out request form and instructions for a 24-hour urine collection for metanephrine and is asked to return when he has completed the collection. You receive the results for the CHEM7 and CBC next morning. The patient returns to the laboratory satellite one week later with the 24-hour urine, but leaves the request forms at home. The phlebotomist calls your office for instructions on how to handle the urine jug while the patient is waiting. After 15 minutes with an angry patient, the phlebotomist receives a copy of the requisition faxed by your office. The metanephrine is ordered and results arrive two days later. You hunt down the laboratory results received a week earlier from the stack of paper on your desk and compare them with the metanephrine results.

Scenario 2

Your associate goes on a vacation cruise in the Caribbean, and you take responsibility for his emergency calls. You receive a call from the laboratory that one of his patients has a phenytoin level of 28 μg/mL, significantly above the 10–20 μg/mL reference range for this laboratory. You vaguely remember a discussion with your associate 6 months ago that this patient is being managed on an anticonvulsant drug above the therapeutic range. You are at home and must go to the office to review the patient's chart.

Scenario 3

You have recently converted your office to electronic laboratory orders and results available through your new electronic medical record system. This system has greatly improved convenient access to laboratory results. You review your computer screen for the CBC ordered 2 days ago on a patient in remission posttreatment for acute myelomonocytic leukemia (AMML). The RBC and WBC counts, the WBC differential, and the RBC indices are all within normal limits. There is a comment in the WBC morphology: "See paper report—not available electronically." Two days later, the paper report arrives. In the WBC morphology field, the comment reads, "One large blast-like mononuclear cell present in smear. Suggest further evaluation and a bone marrow exam." You sigh, "If I had received that information yesterday, the patient would not have been on vacation."

Scenario 4

Your practice has set up a tracking program for following all your hemoglobin A1c results on diabetic patients. This program reminds you of your patient's results so that you can review them before the patient visit. The laboratory performing the test sends out a notice that they will be switching from a method based on immunoassay to a method based on HPLC. A month later, the reminder program indicates that patients are no longer getting their A1c levels. Your patients assure you that they have been to the laboratory. On checking, you find that A1c levels are available from the laboratory and are posted in the electronic medical record. You are confused as to why the error occurred in the reminder program.

Introduction and Overview

Computers play an important role and have had a long history in the clinical laboratory. In most medical centers, the clinical laboratory was the first area outside financial systems to be computerized. The reasons include favorable economics associated with laboratory automation technology and the quantitative nature of most laboratory activity. Early computer efforts focused on delivering results to the clinician, first on paper and later in electronic form. Today, clinicians expect computer systems to provide current and historical patient results in printed form, with Internet access, coupled with electronic orders. The integration of the laboratory with clinical systems is unmatched by any manual system. But this access and availability are very complex examples of interconnected networked systems.

Computerization of the clinical laboratory started in the early 1970s, and by the mid-1980s, about half of laboratories servicing hospitals larger than 200–250 beds had been computerized. In spite of this computerization, most laboratory results, until recently, were delivered to users as paper reports. These laboratory information systems, or LIS, were seldom linked to other computer systems except for billing and then often with magnetic tapes rather than through a real-time interface.

The minicomputer and automated analytical instrumentation made laboratory computerization both economical and necessary. Leonard Skeggs of Case-Western Reserve University (Cleveland, OH) invented the continuous-flow chemistry analyzer in 1950. Technicon Corporation (now a part of Bayer Diagnostics

Corporation) later manufactured this instrument as the AutoAnalyzer. In 1948, the Coulter brothers discovered the principle responsible for counting blood cells. By 1958, the brothers had commercially manufactured their Coulter counter (Coulter is now a part of Beckman Coulter Corporation), automating the complete blood count or CBC. Before the introduction of automated analyzers, laboratory testing relied on manual methods, which were slow and tedious. The usual clinical laboratory produced only a few hundred results per day. By the late 1960s, automated instruments replaced many manual methods in larger laboratories. By the 1970s, an AutoAnalyzer could produce 12 results $\times$ 60 samples per hour, and a Coulter counter could deliver 60 samples $\times$ 7 results per hour. With clinical laboratories producing thousands of individual results a day, data handling had become a significant problem.

By the early 1970s, Digital Equipment Corporation (DEC, now a part of Compaq) sold the first minicomputer for under $1 million. The rapid growth of the clinical laboratories strained data handling, and the annual decrease in the price of computers of 20%–30% made computerization sufficiently attractive. Stand-alone instruments would generate a full-page report (typically for chemistries) or a ticket-like report form (Coulter counter), which was inserted into the patient chart on a self-adhesive form in a shingle-like manner. Paper handling was labor intensive, the shingled reports were chaotic and difficult to follow for trending, and shingles would fall out and disappear when the adhesive aged. Early LISs simply collated results and presented them in a cumulative or tabular format for easy readability. Even though most results were manually entered into the LIS, laboratories justified the cost of the system based on more reliable billing and test reporting. Early LISs maximized the use of expensive hardware but sacrificed flexibility and required a sophisticated central data processing group to handle the frequent changes associated with laboratory testing. Changes, including items such as test definitions, reporting formats, and instrumentation, frequently triggered software changes. As cheaper minicomputer-based systems emerged, software increased in flexibility, and support for the LIS often migrated to laboratory personnel who were often more familiar with managing these changes.

By the early 1980s, mainframe and later crude minicomputer- based clinical information systems, or CISs, started to emerge. Initially the CIS was an extension of the financial system modified to support clinical care. Few of these early systems serviced patient care well. The LIS and CIS largely remained standalone systems for the first 15 years of existence. LIS-to- CIS interfaces were expensive and difficult to implement, and they did not function well. To eliminate the problems of interfacing, some CIS vendors developed a laboratory module. However, vendors found it difficult to dedicate resources to maintain both the clinical and laboratory arenas, and users frequently bought a LIS and a CIS from different vendors for better functionality. Significant deficiencies in displaying laboratory results appeared in early clinical systems. For example, laboratory results were frequently presented and stored as documents rather than individual laboratory results, making retrievals of individual test results difficult.

With the specialization of LISs and CISs, interfacing the two systems became a requirement. By the mid-1980s, Clem McDonald, an internist at the Regenstreif Institute at the Indiana University spearheaded an effort to permit the transfer of laboratory results to downstream clinical systems. This resulted in the development of ASTM (American Society for Testing and Materials) E1238 standard in 1988.[1] The effort to standardize information transfer between systems has grown, resulting in the widening of the scope into the HL7 standards.[2,3] The HL7 standards coordinated and expanded the protocols and rules designed to cover the handling of transactions for electronic orders, financial, administrative, clinical results, and much other information between independent information systems in the clinical environment.

Before discussing the problems associated with interfacing laboratory data, we should discuss (1) the four common types of laboratory data and (2) the relationship between test orders and test results. Because of the rigidity of software associated with many information systems, mismatches between the sending and receiving systems in these two areas are frequently a cause of difficulties.

Types of Laboratory Data

Laboratory Results

Laboratory results can be divided into the following five classes, each with their own characteristics affecting computerization and data transmission.

• Individual numeric answers (e.g., BUN = *12,* sodium = *135*)
• Individual nonnumeric results:
  Single-word answers (e.g., hepatitis B antigen = *negative,* rheumatoid titer = *1:8*)
  Short phrases (e.g., *Platelets are slightly clumped, Results called to floor.*)
• Formatted text (e.g., interpretive reports and free text)
• Progressive multiresult (e.g., microbiology reports)
• FDA-regulated results (blood bank or immunohematology)

It is not surprising that most laboratory and clinical systems handle the first two types of results with few problems. Significant variations and limitations in the handling of formatted text and microbiology reports cause laboratories to use idiosyncrasies of an LIS to report these more specialized situations. This, in turn, causes problems when results are transferred to another system, even one designed by the same vendor. Because of their time-dependent and progressively changing nature, microbiology reports are particularly complex. Blood bank portions of the LIS are regulated by the FDA as a class I medical device since they are responsible for checking the distribution of correct blood products to patients, tracking information with regard to collected blood products, and long-term retention of transfusion and patient information.

Transferring laboratory information from the LIS to the CIS is complicated by the differences in the storage and presentation of data. We will briefly summarize issues that can affect each of the data types when transmitted between computer systems. For convenience, we will refer to two types of reporting formats. The first, often referred to as the interim format, presents a single result on a single line, usually in the format

Test name, Test result, Reference range, Other flags/Comments

The second, often called the cumulative report format, presents results in a tabular manner similar to a Lotus or Excel spreadsheet. Typically, the first column (or row) is the test name and the remaining columns (or rows) are filled in with test results.

Individual Numeric Results

Numeric results are probably the most common format used in the laboratory, and most systems today handle numbers in a consistent manner. Numeric results are checked by the LIS to meet normal limits, critical values, intrapatient variability, and so on. The LIS takes actions depending on the outcome of these checks. For example, if the number is not credible, it asks the laboratory technologist to reenter it, or if the result is outside the reference range, it sets the abnormal result flag. Numbers stored in a computer are in the form of either integers ($\ldots, -2, -1, 0, +1, +2, \ldots$) or real numbers (e.g., $1.016* 10^6$). Most computers have limitations on the size of numbers in either notation, but usually this is not a practical problem. For example, a very large integer number, such as 1,283,575, may be rounded off to 1,283,000.

Two problems frequently occur with numeric results. First, many systems report clinical laboratory results using a table-like format able to display cumulative results in a very dense manner. The column width used in these tables limits the number of characters displayed. For example, if this limit is 8 characters, the number 1,283,575, containing 9 characters, does not fit. When such results cannot be displayed, most systems provide alternatives for the user to retrieve the results, but the extra steps may be inconvenient and skipped by the user. A second problem can occur when numeric results are sent across an interface (although it happens rarely): the sending system fails to send the result in the format expected by the receiving system and format conversion does not occur (e.g., the LIS sends a result in scientific notation, but the clinical system expects an integer). To avoid this, the sending and receiving computers require close coordination to make the presentation and user interaction acceptable.

Individual Nonnumeric Results

Both single-word and preprogrammed or canned short phrases are handled similarly by computers and have similar problems. Examples of single-word results include *Positive, Negative,* and titers such as *1:8.* Examples of short phrase results include *Presence of spherocytosis* and *Occasional clumping of platelets seen.* If an information system presents single-word results in a table, column width limitations similar to those for numeric results can occur. In a cumulative report with an 8-character limit, the result *Positive* fits, but the word *Hemolyzed* does not. The interim report format is likely to be more forgiving for single-word results, but longer phrases require that the computer system chop up the phrase into two or more lines.

Without numeric properties, a computer system cannot perform as many checks on nonnumeric results as it can on numeric results. Since nonnumeric results are discrete phrases, they lack the mathematical properties of integers or real numbers. For example, antibodies consist of a set of normal, borderline, and abnormal titers. These titers are stepwise rather than continuous and are usually treated as text results. Flagging abnormal nonnumeric values requires that the computer compare each result with a table, a feature that may be absent in some systems.

Formatted and Free Text

Interpretations of laboratory results in the form of free or formatted text create additional challenges. From a data-handling standpoint, text is a variable string consisting of words separated by carriage returns, tabs, indentation, pagination, and so on, usually to improve the readability of a report. The most common formatting technique is paragraphing. Another example is the creation of tables using tabs, indents, and lines. For humans, formatted text is relatively easy to enter and comprehend.

Unfortunately, a computer has great difficulty in the storage, retrieval, and management of this kind of data. The unstructured nature of text allows substantial ambiguity in its content and formatting. At the simplest level, retention of text formatting between computer systems is difficult, since the sizes of displayed characters, the length of a line, and the number of lines per page can all vary from computer to computer. Web browsers partially resolve this problem by requiring the sender to specify formatting information for lines, paragraphs, and pages. Unfortunately, older systems may not have such capabilities, requiring programmers to spend large amounts of time to resolve differences during the implementation of interface software. A laboratory carefully formats a complex interpretive report in a lab system using carriage returns and other devices, but this formatting is lost when the report is transmitted to a browser-based data warehouse where the entire report is a single block of text. With the removal from the report of carriage return separators, the text may be unreadable.

Few, if any, clinical information systems at this time can "read free text" to extract pertinent information. Research is progressing on natural language processors, which will read narrative text from dictated summaries and extract data. Most current systems require users to explicitly specify the information in a structured manner and from a restricted vocabulary. For this reason, any abnormal flags appearing on a dictated summary usually require that the narrator specify the flag.

Progressively Changing Results

Results that progressively change over time are the most complex and pose special problems. Clinical microbiology is the best example. A microbiology result typically consists of three parts. A preliminary examination (e.g., a gram stain) is usually followed by a culture. If the cultures result in growth of one or more pathogenic organisms, antibiotic sensitivity testing is performed. At least three characteristics of microbiology results distinguish them from other result types. These characteristics challenge the transmission of results between systems. First, culture results may be updated multiple times. A report of no growth at 24 hours may be followed by positive growth on subsequent days. Each update requires the coordination of the sending and receiving system so that results are synchronized. Second, these results may remain pending for as long as several weeks (e.g., for tuberculosis mycobacterium). Third, antibiotic sensitivities are ordered only when the organism has been identified. Therefore, the receiving system will be required to link new results to older finalized results.

The complexity of microbiology results usually requires both LISs and clinical systems to handle them separately from other laboratory results. The CIS handles microbiology results through one of two mechanisms. The first approach simply accepts preformatted reports from the LIS and displays them without regard to format. Since most clinical systems already have the ability to accept transcribed reports, this approach is simple to implement. The sending LIS must be equipped to retransmit all relevant parts of the updated report each time. For example, the preliminary examination and organism identifications must be resent when the sensitivities are added. Most clinical systems avoid the use of preformatted reports because they cannot perform actions based on such data.

CIS systems today prefer to accept microbiology reports in a more structured data format. The data format transmits results in a manner preserving the data collected by the laboratory. As a compromise, some systems accept the preformatted report for displaying the result to the clinician and data format for processing by the CIS. Systems receiving results only in the data format require local software to manipulate and link all portions of the result to display the final report, regardless of when the results were received. Problems are encountered when the receiving system expects the LIS to integrate clinical information with its data. For example, a positive *Staphylococcus epidermis* result on a skin culture may be quite significant in an immunocompromised or burn patient but unimportant otherwise. Since the LIS frequently does not have clinical information, it cannot determine significance.

Many clinical systems use microbiology data to create antibiotic sensitivity matrices. These matrices list organisms on one axis and antibiotics on the second axis. The principal advantage of this approach is that the clinician is able to immediately identify appropriate antibiotics to administer to a patient infected with multiple organisms. Such an approach requires organism names and antibiotic names to be carefully synchronized in both the CIS and LIS. Synchronization problems may occur, for example, when new antibiotics are introduced, organisms change names, or one antibiotic sensitivity test substitutes for others in the same family (e.g., penicillin is replaced by ampicillin on one system but not the other).

TABLE 4.1 Two-level test request.

Order level 2	Chemistry profile, 7 tests
Order level 1	Sodium
(single test)	Potassium
	Chloride
	Carbon dioxide (CO_2)
	Glucose
	Blood urea nitrogen (BUN)
	Creatinine

FDA-Regulated Results

The most common FDA-regulated results are immunohematology or blood bank results. Blood bank results include all information related to testing for blood transfusion, including blood typing, blood compatibility testing, and management and administration of blood products. Unlike other clinical laboratory software, the FDA has classified software handling the dispensation of blood products as a class III medical device, the most rigorous classification the FDA applies. In addition to stringent vendor requirements, this requires any institution using blood bank software to test any implementation extensively. Blood bank information systems may be integrated into the LIS or may operate as a stand-alone system. The CIS may receive transfusion results via their interface to an LIS. Real-time interfaces between clinical systems and a central blood bank supplier are uncommon because suppliers are reluctant to perform the software testing needed and because such systems lack the patient information needed to allow the CIS to receive results. Blood types and transfusion history may also be manually entered into either the laboratory or the clinical system. The laboratory often does not have immediate feedback from a clinical service that transfusion has occurred. In such instances, the computer tags the blood product as "presumed transfused" if the unit is not returned to the laboratory within a defined window (e.g., 24 hours). Consequently, clinicians will not know with certainty whether the patient was transfused.

Relationship of Test Requests (or Orders) to Test Results

For most laboratory tests, clinicians can order tests in one of four ways. (1) In the simplest form, a *single order* translates to a single test result. For example, a creatinine request translates to a single creatinine result of 0.7 μg/dL. (2) In another common relationship, a *test panel or battery* translates into many results. For example, a *CBC* reports 8 numbers (hemoglobin, hematocrit, MCV, MCHC, MCH, RBC, WBC, platelet count); a request for a seven-test chemistry panel or *basic metabolic panel* generates seven chemistry results (sodium, potassium, chloride, carbon dioxide, glucose, creatinine, and blood urea nitrogen). For convenience, we refer to this as a two-level test request (Table 4.1). (3) A three-level test request (Table 4.2) combines several two-level tests. We refer to this as a multiple panel

TABLE 4.2 Three-level test request.

Order level 3 (multiple panels)	CBC with differential	
Order level 2 (battery)	CBC	WBC differential
Order level 1 (single test)	Hemoglobin	Neutrophils
	Hematocrit	Lymphocytes
	WBC count	Monocytes
	RBC count	Eosinophils
	MCV	Basophils
	MCHC	
	MCH	
	Platelet count	

TABLE 4.3 Four-level test request.

Order level 4	Admission profile			
Order level 3	CBC with differential		Chemistry profile, 7 tests	Coagulation profile
Order level 2	CBC	WBC differential		
Order level 1	Hemoglobin	Neutrophils	Sodium	Thrombin time
	Hematocrit	Lymphocytes	Potassium	Prothrombin time
	WBC count	Monocytes	Chloride	APTT
	RBC count	Eosinophils	CO_2	
	MCV	Basophils	Glucose	
	MCHC		BUN	
	MCH		Creatinine	
	Platelet count			

or battery. A common three-level test is CBC with differential, which combines the two-level tests CBC and WBC differential. Microbiology tests can be described as a specialized three-level structure to be covered later. (4) A four-level structure (Table 4.3) is less commonly incorporated as a unique entity within most information systems for laboratory results, but it is frequently utilized within medical practices, usually in the form of an *order set*. An order set bundles a number of individual laboratory orders, most frequently to fill the needs of a specific care protocol (e.g., an inpatient admissions profile). The advantage of a four-level structure is that it simplifies maintenance of tables used to define tests in the information systems and may enable users to selectively delete and add tests more conveniently.

Knowledge of the ordering relationships can be highly useful to the receiving system for displaying results. Receiving systems may cluster related results using locally maintained tables (e.g., cluster all chemistry together in the order specified by a table of chemistry tests). Alternatively, the receiving system can cluster tests using ordering information. This information is sent with results by most LISs. The danger with using tables in the receiving system is that changes in the LIS must be carefully coordinated with the CIS. If a chemistry test's name is changed in the LIS, for example, it may appear in the miscellaneous test area in the CIS with other ungrouped tests rather than in the chemistry area, making the result harder to find or missed by a busy clinician.

To ensure that results are properly identified, orders and results are often linked through specimen numbers. These are transaction numbers issued by either the LIS or the CIS to identify a particular test order. This specimen number may also be bar-coded. Bar codes applied to specimen containers for positive identification greatly reduce the chance of errors associated with misidentification. Although standards have been created for specimen bar codes by ASTM[4] and the National Committee for Clinical Laboratory Standards,[5] incompatibilities between systems often prevent the application of bar codes on specimens being generated by a foreign system (i.e, the bar code used by an LIS must be generated by the LIS). It is hoped that future standards efforts will enable bar codes to be used across systems.

Interface Architectures

To interconnect to other information systems, most vendors have designed software interface modules to link external vendor systems. For most LIS systems, vendors have divided interfaces into those that support the receipt of orders from a foreign system (orders interface) and those that transmit results to an external system (results interface). From both a technical and a marketing perspective, the division of systems into orders and results makes sense. Most interfaces are designed around the HL7 standard[2,3] and its formal subset ASTM 1238,[1] which provide a formal structure for sending and receiving laboratory transactions. These standards have greatly reduced vendor variations in interface design. These standards have also resulted in the appearance of interface engines, i.e., software and hardware packages with toolkits dedicated to handling and transmitting HL7 messages. Interface engines permit information systems to accept inputs from and send outputs to multiple systems (e.g., one-to-many and many-to-one interfaces). Since they do not require the detailed development of software from scratch, these devices have been used to decrease the time and costs of interfaces.

In spite of standards, the complexity and costs of implementing LIS/CIS interfaces remains high. For example, a major LIS vendor charges about $15,000 for each results or orders interface and requires 1 to 3 months to complete the task. Therefore, a complete LIS/CIS orders and results interface could cost more than $60,000, assuming that an equal amount is charged by the CIS vendor and excluding the expenses the customer incurs in implementing the interface. Generally, an LIS results interface is simpler to implement than an orders interface. Because interface implementations are personnel intensive, there have not been significant decreases in the vendor pricing of interfaces over the last 10 years, even with the rapid increases in their sales.

Interfaces can be divided into three functional units. The first translates the internal data representation from or to a data representation understood by the receiving system (translator). The second packages or formats the transmission into

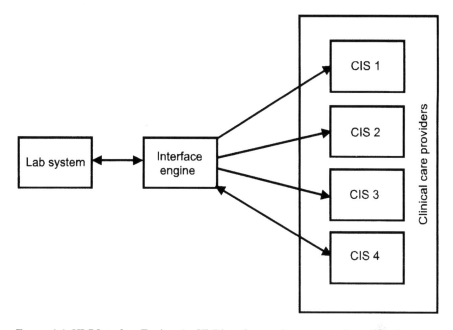

FIGURE 4.1. HL7 Interface Engine. An HL7 interface engine connects four clinical systems to an LIS. CIS # 1, CIS # 2 and CIS # 3 receive results from the LIS through the interface engine. CIS # 4 receive results and sends orders through the interface engine.

or from units understood by the receiving system (formatter). In most cases, both sides must perform some translation and formatting. The third functional unit transmits or receives the information using the underlying hardware or computer network (transmitter/receiver). The translator is likely to be different for every hospital since it depends on local terminology and work flow. The formatter is specific to each LIS vendor/CIS vendor pair. The transmitter/receiver depends on the underlying hardware and network used by the CIS/LIS.

An HL7 interface engine connects four clinical systems to an LIS. CIS 1, CIS 2 and CIS 3 receive results from the LIS through the interface engine. CIS 4 receive results and sends orders through the interface engine (Figure 4.1).

Results Interfaces

To implement a results interface, software development starts at the lowest level and works up to a more complex level. A network connection between the LIS and CIS must first be established, followed by development of the receiver and transmitter software. Once a connection exists, the formatter(s) between the LIS and CIS must be developed. Finally, the user must identify differences between the source and the destination fields and how they should be translated. For test names, this consists of a table with LIS and CIS test names. In the simplest case, the LIS interface software takes the LIS test name and translate it to the CIS test name through the table. Other more complex translations can also be made (e.g., translation of results to/from SI units or the formatting of microbiology free text).

To reduce site-specific translations, some have advocated the use of the standardized laboratory test nomenclature LOINC (logical observation identifiers names and codes).[6] In this approach, the laboratory or LIS translates from its internal nomenclature to LOINC. The CIS receives the LOINC nomenclature and translates it for local presentation. This two-step translation process is more complex if there is only a single sending and receiving interface. In the situation where an LIS interfaces to multiple CISs or an CIS interfaces to multiple LISs, maintenance of translation tables can be substantially reduced.

In an environment without an orders interface, most LISs send results with little consideration for the receiving system. Usually the receiving system takes full responsibility for accepting the result and storing it properly. The only complication is when the results in the receiving system (usually a CIS) are updated by the LIS. This occurs routinely and frequently with microbiology results. It also occurs when the laboratory updates a test result (e.g., a corrected result) or when the LIS sends test statuses prior to the final result. In such a situation, the receiving system often identifies the result by patient name and collection time/date or by a unique transaction (or serial) number. The transaction number approach is better since it is possible for the collection time/date to be changed if that has been entered in error.

Orders Interfaces

Unlike results interfaces, orders interfaces require substantial synchronization between an initiating event—the order—and the closure of the event—the completion of all orders with results. Without the linkage of the orders to results, the laboratory simply returns results without closing orders, and the physician is unable to determine which orders are complete or require other action. The linkage of the order to results greatly complicates the interface. In most systems, a unique transaction number is required for the tracking to operate properly. When a CIS issues a order, it also issues a transaction number, which is sent along with the order to the LIS. The LIS accepts this number and appends an identifying prefix to make it unique. Alternatively, it issues another transaction number and links it to the CIS transaction number. From this time forward, both systems link the order and associated results to the transaction number(s). In this way, any data parameter can change, including the patient number, and both systems can track the result appropriately. If the links between orders and results are lost, the LIS and CIS may both have pending transactions, requiring the system managers to evaluate the pending events and close them manually, a tedious task. Alternatively, some systems simply cancel open orders after a certain time has elapsed. Even if this procedure works, it has the disadvantage of being sloppy since it does not identify the cause of the open events and is an invitation for errors.

Common Interface Problem Areas

Even with the best-designed interface, problems frequently occur when sending laboratory data. For purposes of this chapter, the problems are divided into two major classifications. The first class of problems is those caused by the lack of coordination between the sending and the receiving system, at either the personnel or the system design level. At the personnel level, problems occur because of the lack of knowledge of limitations between the sending and receiving system and are usually avoidable through education and experience. At the system level, problems occur because designers omit the detection and conversion of incompatible data. The second class are problems usually triggered by random events that result in the disruption and/or loss of synchronization between the sending and receiving systems. These problems are often difficult to detect in an automated fashion, and overcoming them may require complex designs. Over the past three to four years, we have observed the following problem areas when transmitting data from the LIS to a CIS.

Formatting Problems Associated with Data Coordination

Length Limitations of Test Names

The LIS used at the University of Washington allows test names of 35 characters. Some downstream systems are limited to 24 characters. It is important that test names be limited to around 24 characters or be defined in a way that truncation does not affect meaning. For example, the test names "Hepatitis C virus quantitation by PCR" and "Hepatitis C virus quantitation by ELISA" would both appear as "Hepatitis C virus quanti," which results in a loss of information for someone trying to interpret results.

Length Limitations of Results

Systems reporting in a columnar fashion ("cumulative report format") has column width limits. This is usually arbitrary and around eight to ten characters. The wider field size permits the display of complex results at the expense of displaying fewer events. Results longer than the column width usually will not display and therefore inconvenience the user by requiring multiple accesses (e.g., mouse clicks) to review the result. The clinician may bypass the result lookup.

Formatted text may also have length limitations. For example, sending a 2000-character report causes unpredictable problems in a system limited to 500 characters. In the worst case, the report may be truncated or lost.

Order of Tests in Batteries or Panels

Downstream systems may not preserve the reporting order or grouping of tests as used in the LIS. For example, an anemia panel consisting of a hemoglobin and a

B12 grouped together in the LIS may be split to separate chemistry and hematology headers. If order or grouping is important, changes may be required in the formatting of the downstream system.

Variable Handling of Blocks of Formatted Text in Reports

Downstream computer systems differ in the way they handle blocks of text, and result formatting can be unpredictable. For example, systems using Internet Web browser technology ignore line breaks and run everything into a single block of text. This is because the number of characters displayed on a single line depends on the size of the letters and the size of the display window. Likewise, the user may be forced to view the actual results in a location separated from a table if the results do not fit. Shorter results may be broken into several short lines. A large block of text may even be truncated.

Restrictions on the Use of Special Characters

Characters other than uppercase and lowercase letters and numbers (A–Z, a–z, 0–9) may be displayed unpredictably, particularly in systems using Internet Web browsers, where a special character in the sending system can be interpreted as a formatting character in the receiving system. For example, !, <, >, and & have special meanings for Internet browsers and computer system interfaces. Browsers should be tested for proper display of test names and results containing these characters for proper translation. Complicating this task is that all versions of browsers in use should be checked (e.g., Netscape major and minor versions of 3.X, 4.X, and versions for PC, Macintosh, and Unix; Explorer 3.X, 4.0, 4.5 5.0, 5.1, 5.5, and versions for PC and Macintosh; and so on).

Problems Caused by Loss of Data Synchronization

Recovery from a Computer Crash

Recovery from an unexpected computer failure is among the most challenging tasks for any software designer. This task is made more difficult when two or more computer systems from different vendors are networked together since each system must establish their relationship to each linked system. For a results interface, reestablishing the relationships between systems can usually be performed by resending all results after a certain time period. Most systems sending results save a sequential log of results sent to downstream systems along with a time stamp of each transaction. To ensure that all results are sent, a system must simply pick a time point before the failure. Resent results can overwrite previous results or be ignored by the receiving system.

Synchronizing an orders and results interface can be substantially more complex. The following sequence creates problems. A physician places an order in the CIS, but the order has not been transmitted to the LIS. The CIS aborts suddenly, but the specimen is collected and sent to the laboratory. The laboratory performs the test without an CIS order. The LIS sends a result back to the CIS. The CIS determines that this is an unsolicited test request generated without an CIS order. The pending CIS order is received when the CIS recovers, resulting in an unneeded order being sent to the LIS. Usually clearing this type of error requires human intervention to identify and delete the duplicate orders.

Changed or Corrected Results

Changes in data occurring in either sending or receiving information systems require a corresponding change in the other linked systems. A change in data in a receiving station will usually force a manual update of the sending system. In most cases, a sending system can update a downstream system when results are changed. Representative tests and tests in which changes in results are common or anticipated should be tested to show whether the corrections are reported accurately and clearly. Idiosyncratic behavior can also exist in interfaces. For example, changes in test demographics, including ordering time and date, do not result in updates in clinical systems in some interfaces. Changes in these elements require that the user delete the original test request/result and reorder/result all elements.

Synchronization of Microbiology Results

Because microbiology requires frequent updates as organisms are identified and sensitivities are performed, downstream systems must use specialized software for reporting. Therefore, microbiology results must be tested independently of other laboratory reporting. Another problem area is that antibiotic/organism sensitivity matrices may require maintenance whenever new organisms or antibiotics are encountered.

Other Issues

Trending/Tracking of Results

Changing test mnemonics, test characteristics, or reference ranges can affect trending and results tracking/extract programs in downstream systems. Some systems can link similar tests (e.g., hemoglobin A1c by HPLC and hemoglobin A1c by ELISA). Such linking usually requires manual intervention somewhere by system maintenance personnel. In other cases, changes are required in the programs performing the trending or tracking function. Since most linkages are performed through interactions between support personnel on different systems, failures occur most often when communications fail with new systems or new support personnel. Linking of similar tests may not be possible in some information systems, presenting another level of difficulty.

Flags and Alerts

Abnormal flags are issued by an LIS on most tests, but the reference ranges of flags are usually based on the characteristics of the entire population serviced by the laboratory. They may cause excessive or insufficient flagging for specialized populations or for an individual patient (e.g., an epileptic on an elevated phenytoin dose). Most clinical systems simply take the LIS flag and transfer it to their database. Ideally, abnormal flagging should be individualized, either by the clinician entering the parameters into an CIS or through recognition of appropriate clinical situations by the CIS.

LIS may not be able to flag some tests, properly. For example, a positive urine culture with 100 colonies of *E. coli* should be flagged in an immunocompromised transplant patient but could be ignored for a primary care patient. Since most LISs do not have accurate clinical diagnoses for most patients, proper flagging is difficult.

Laboratory handling of alerts have similar problems. LISs often require that the system distinguish between two methods or instruments for workflow reasons, even though both sets of results should be treated together. It is necessary for the reports generating alerts to be aware of all closely related tests so that the alert recognizes whether or not the appropriate patient care conditions have been met.

Discussion of Introductory Scenarios

Scenario 1

Unfortunately, patients do appear in the laboratory without paperwork indicating what tests are being requested. In most cases, the phlebotomist or the clerk must make telephone calls to the ordering physician for this information, resulting in the patient waiting and wasted time at the laboratory and in the physician's office. Even if the practitioner or nurse is available to provide this information immediately, further delays result if he/she must refer to the paper chart. On the laboratory side, the clerk receiving the urine metanephrine request will have difficulty tying the order to the blood tests ordered several days earlier. This results in paper reports arriving at the physician's office separately.

An electronic interface between a CIS and an LIS for physician orders eliminates the need for a telephone call when a patient arrives without a paper requisition. Too often, however, organizations eliminate all paper and rely entirely on the interface. Although this approach appears efficient, it fails if one or more parts of a complex computer system are unavailable. An LIS by itself has about 40 hours of downtime annually if it operates with 99.5% reliability. If other information systems and their interconnections each have similar reliability, the annual expected downtime triples. Unlike the situation where only a few patients forget their paperwork, a nonfunctioning computer system requires that the laboratory call on every patient for orders, creating much added work for the clinician and laboratory as well as the potential for unhappy patients. Paper requisitions provide an inexpensive backup system for the electronic system. The electronic system complements this by eliminating difficulties associated with the occasional problem patient. Electronic results can also provide the clinician with consolidated laboratory results of tests performed on separate days even if the orders are not properly linked.

Scenario 2

For most laboratory systems, patient result flagging continues to be driven by global (e.g., institutional) parameters rather than patient-specific ones. Although the drug response of an individual patient can vary by a factor of 10, reference ranges in an LIS do not reflect this, resulting in unnecessary calls for patients chronically dosed in the "toxic range." Ideally, flagging should be performed by information systems with sufficient clinical information to provide the patient care provider with adjustable flagging parameters. At the simplest level, the patient care provider can set flagging parameters manually. Better yet are systems that review results using rules and patient-specific information. As electronic medical record systems become more comprehensive, such capabilities will become more sophisticated.

Scenario 3

Matching all the requirements of both the sending and the receiving systems can be challenging. One of the more common problems is the limit on the size of a columnar display. By putting results in multiple columns (also referred to as the cumulative or spreadsheet format), it is possible to increase the density of displayed results and aid in trend analysis. Most systems, however, do not dynamically adjust the width of columns to fit the data. When some LISs send a result wider than the displayable width on the CIS, they abort the result and ask the user to refer to the paper report. Other systems truncate the report. Finally, systems may hold the report in a separate area and require the user to navigate to that screen. This approach is preferable over the first two in that the full report can be displayed. However, a novice user may not be aware of how to retrieve the result, especially if the navigation process is not intuitive. Both the laboratory and clinical systems support personnel must be aware of display limitations. Most important, users must also be trained to recognize when information is missing so that they can retrieve it in an appropriate manner.

Scenario 4

This physician is having problems with the laboratory changing its test mnemonics. Updates were not made in the clinical information system's tracking and alert programs to follow the laboratory changes. Since it was rapid and convenient, the laboratory had been using a manual point-of-care test (POCT) for performing hemoglobin A1c tests. Since the volume had increased to over 1000 tests per month, the five minutes of tech time and the $10 per cartridge had started to challenge both bookkeeping and tech time. The laboratory continued to provide the POCT to the endocrinologists who needed the rapid turnaround and performed overnight testing by HLPC on an automated instrument for other users. These changes were passed to the clinical systems personnel. Unfortunately, the alerts were being maintained by a separate group of clinicians who did not receive the communications.

References

1. ASTM designation E1238–97, standard specification for transferring clinical laboratory data messages between independent computer systems, *1999 Annual Book of ASTM Standards,* Vol. 14.01, pp. 100–179. American Society for Testing and Materials, Philadelphia, 1999.
2. Beeler, GW. HL7 version 3—An object-oriented methodology for collaborative standards development. *Int J Med Inf* 1998 Feb;48(1–3):151–61.
3. Van Hentenryck K. Health Level Seven: Shedding light on HL7's Version 2.3 standard. *Healthcare Informatics* 1997 Mar;14(3):74.
4. ASTM designation E1466–92, standard specification for use of bar codes on specimen tubes in the clinical laboratory, *1999 Annual Book of ASTM Standards,* Vol. 14.01, pp. 451–453. American Society for Testing and Materials, Philadelphia, 1999.
5. Chou D, Davis R, Moss P, and Stevens T. *Laboratory Automation: Bar Codes for Specimen Container Identification; Standard Auto2A.* National Committee for Clinical Laboratory Standards, Wayne, PA, volume 20, number 19, October, 2000.
6. Forrey AW, McDonald CJ, DeMoor G, Huff SM, Leavelle D, Leland D, Fiers T, Charles L, Griffin B, Stalling F, Tullis A, Hutchins K, Baenziger J. Logical observation identifier names and codes (LOINC) database: A public use set of codes and names for electronic reporting of clinical laboratory test results. *Clin Chem* 1996 Jan;42(1):81–90.

5
Importing Images

BRENT K. STEWART, PH.D., ET AL.

Scenario

At the University of Washington Academic Medical Center, a primary care physician logs into MINDscape (a Web-based electronic medical record) from her office and proceeds to the results of a recent radiological examination for one of her patients. Presented with an HTML list of radiology examinations (Figure 5.1), she selects one by clicking on its hyperlink. This takes her to the page with the radiology report she wants (Figure 5.2). On the report page is an icon representing the hyperlink to the associated set of radiological images for that exam. Selecting this hyperlink brings up a new multiframed window (Figure 5.3) that includes all image series generated during the exam, as well as associated patient and exam demographics, including the report. In addition, the radiologist has created a subset of relevant images with text and graphical annotations indicating the region of concern.

Still uncertain about how a specific finding cited in the radiology report will affect treatment, she phones the reading radiologist with her query. The radiologist, after answering this call, logs into either a display workstation in the radiology department, his office computer, or his home computer, and they review the images together over the network. Once the on-line interactive conference has concluded, the radiologist saves the newly annotated image as a "significant" image and continues with his work. The primary care physician, having refreshed her browser window, selects the newly annotated image and either copies it into a patient summary document, stores it in a teaching file, or e-mails it to a colleague for consultation.

This scenario appears rather seamless, but it is made possible by a vast matrix of people, computers, networks, standards, and software processes behind the scenes. This chapter describes the processes that make this scenario a reality at the University of Washington Academic Medical Centers. The data flow diagram describing the flow of information is presented in Figure 5.4.

Background

Since Wilhelm Conrad Roentgen's day, film has been the traditional method for capturing and displaying information in radiological imaging. This method has served the discipline well; screen–film radiography can achieve exquisite spatial resolution, and it provides a reasonably dynamic range of optical densities for display of image contrast. Film is a jack-of-all-trades: it serves as image acquisition,

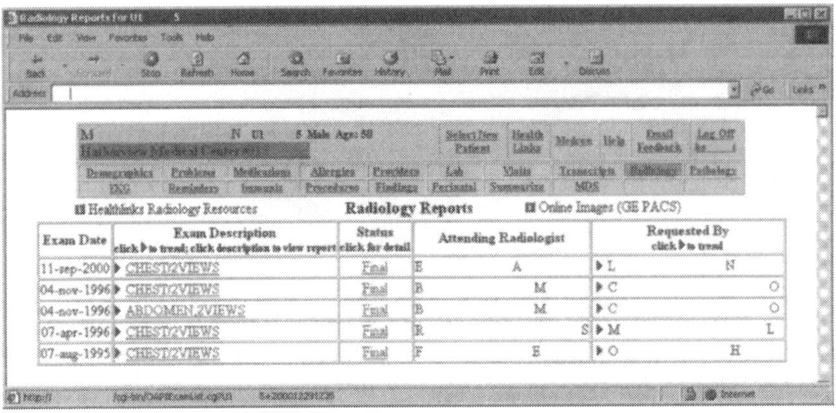

FIGURE 5.1. List of radiology reports for a dummy test patient using MINDscape. A list of all radiology exams in the PACS can be directly accessed through the "Online Images" icon button above the radiology report list for patient. A specific radiology examination image set can be accessed directly through the individual icon button for each report or through the radiology report.

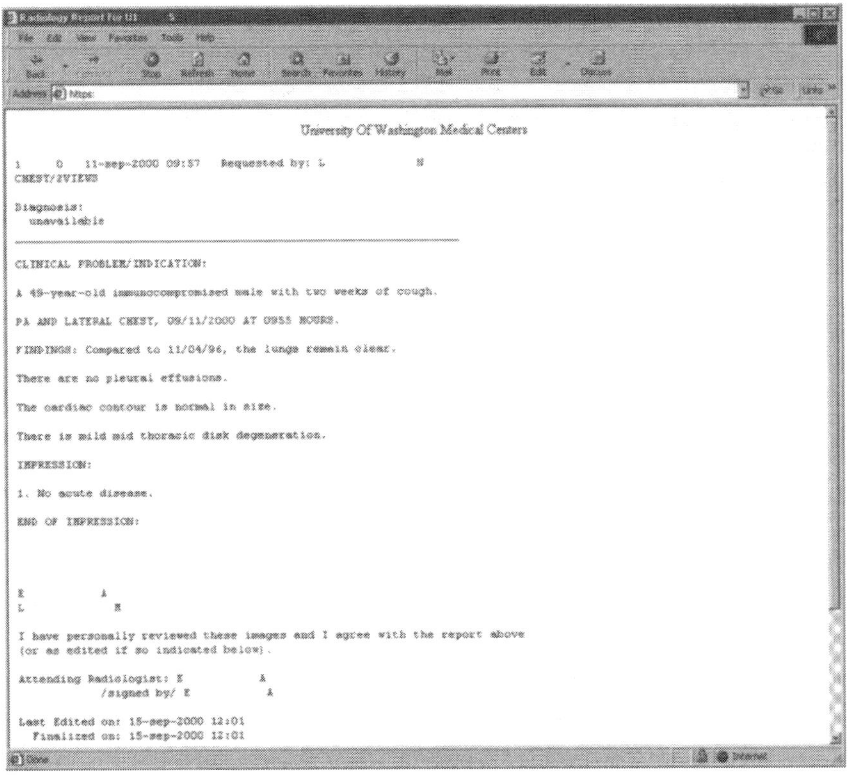

FIGURE 5.2. Test patient radiology report for the specified PA and Lateral (Chest 2 views — CHEST/2V) exam accessed through the exam report hyperlink in Figure 5.1.

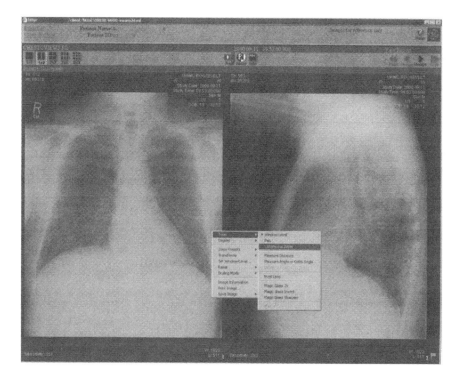

FIGURE 5.3. PA chest image displayed for the dummy test patient created by the PACS Web server and associated with the exam report hyperlink shown in Figure 5.2. This image and the associated report in Figure 5.2 are linked through the RIS exam accession number (1xxxxx0).

display, and storage devices. No other medium can compare with film's multitasking capability, even though film is by no means optimal for every solitary task.

The greatest attraction of film is that it is analog. We live in an analog world; our everyday experience is continuous, not discrete. Film is very user friendly. We humans are very tactile creatures, and touching objects makes them somehow more "real" to us. There is nothing in the digital world quite like the solid feel of paging through a good book or passing family snapshots around the kitchen table. The primary mode of ordering radiology examinations is still through paper requisition (and don't forget to enter that ICD-9 code).

However, film has some severe disadvantages that are becoming increasingly problematic in a busy radiology service: repeat exposures are frequent; films are not immediately available for review; it is necessary to properly dispose of the by-products of film processing; a film cannot be spontaneously viewed simultaneously anywhere within an institution, the country, or the world. The film library is often the bottleneck in the clinical information workflow constituting an interpretive and consultative medical imaging service. Lost, misplaced, and misappropriated films are a constant problem that not only frustrates radiologists and referring physicians

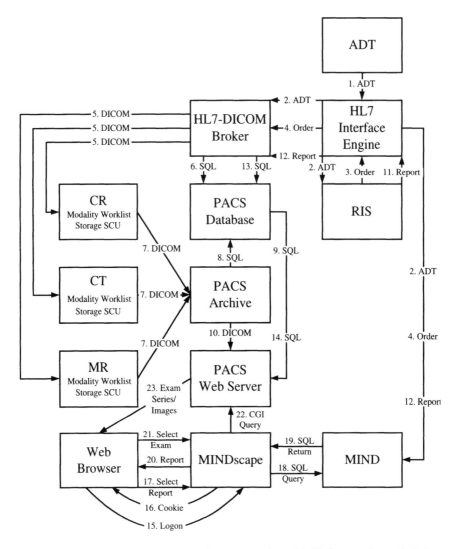

FIGURE 5.4. Workflow and data migration process for a PACS from patient admission through primary care physician review of the images from the PACS Web server. Each step in this process is labeled with a sequential number and described in the text. CR = computed radiography. CT = computed tomography. MR = magnetic resonance imaging.

but also compromises the quality of patient care. We will never have a "cradle to grave" medical record that uses paper and film.

The widespread adoption of electronic radiology (e.g., Picture Archiving and Communication Systems, or PACS[1,2]) is inevitable, just as electric lighting, radio, and television has been. All new technologies when invented, developed, and marketed go through an adoption life cycle. The percent of society adopting the technology over time generally describes a sigmoidal-shaped curve, ironically similar to the contrast curve of radiography film. The evolution of technology adoption follows a fairly predictable course. First the innovators (2%–4%) break new technological ground. Next come the visionaries, or the early adopters (12%–14%). Between the early adopters and the early majority lies the chasm, where many technological innovations become mired or expire. The PACS chasm has been bridged recently, and the early majority (34%) has begun to implement electronic radiology. The late majority (34%) and the laggards (16%) bring up the rear. We are not too far along the technology adoption curve of PACS, but the next few years will see rapid deployment of these systems. Eventually electronic radiology will be fully adopted as the standard for patient care, the laggards will finally capitulate, and film will be relegated to the silver reclamation bin.

Scenario Process Decomposition

The scenario process begins with patient demographic information being transmitted as Health Level 7 (HL7) messages from the Admission-Discharge-Transfer (ADT) system (Figure 5.4) when the patient arrives at the medical center as either an inpatient or outpatient (step 1). These messages are routed through an interface engine that buffers, reformats, and retransmits these messages to one or many downstream target HL7 systems (step 2). The ADT information is used by the Radiology Information System (RIS) to provide authoritative data for the population of patient demographic fields in the RIS when patient examinations are scheduled into the system through either manual entry of radiology exam requisitions or electronic order entry. The scheduling of an exam into the RIS triggers the RIS to transmit an HL7 order message to the HL7 interface engine where it is buffered (step 3). Copies of the RIS order HL7 message are then transmitted to the Medical Information Networked Database (MIND, the electronic medical record database) and to an HL7-DICOM broker (step 4), which also received (in step 2) a copy of the ADT message from the HL7 interface engine.

The HL7-DICOM (Digital Imaging and Communications in Medicine) broker is itself simply another interface engine that takes in HL7 messages and transmits DICOM messages, in this case DICOM Modality Worklist information (step 5), to the imaging modalities (e.g., Computed Tomography) for inclusion with the created images. The function of the DICOM Modality Worklist Service Class is to push relevant patient demographic and scheduled exam information to the imaging modalities. At the imaging modalities, the radiology technologists simply select scheduled patient exams from a worklist, rather than rely on manual entry of this information, which is prone to transposition and other types of input error. The HL7-DICOM broker database also communicates with the PACS database (step 6) through structured query language (SQL) transactions. This patient and exam information is required by the PACS database in order to marry this information with the images (step 8) from the modality once they are received by the PACS archive through DICOM storage service class messages after exam completion (step 7). Once the exam is complete and the exam images reside in the PACS archive, the text (step 9) and image (step 10) information are transferred to the PACS Web server where the images are compressed and a universal resource locator (URL) is assigned to each exam.

When the radiology report is finalized through electronic signature, a copy is sent to the HL7 interface engine (step 11) and forwarded to the HL7-DICOM broker (step 12). The HL7–DICOM broker in turn forwards this copy to the PACS database (step 13) where it is entered and copied to the PACS Web server (step 14).

It is at this point that the user (e.g., the primary care physician in her office) logs into MINDscape through a Web browser (step 15) that supports encryption of the data stream passing to and from it. MINDscape returns an encrypted cookie (authentication token) to the browser (step 16) for subsequent queries to MINDscape. The user selects the desired report (step 17, Figure 5.1) from the list of patient radiological examinations in MINDscape. MINDscape sends an SQL request to the Medical Information Networked Database (MIND) to return the selected radiology report (step 18). MIND returns the correct radiological exam report to MINDscape (step 19). MINDscape returns the selected report to the browser in hypertext markup language (HTML) format (step 20; see Figure 5.2). The user elects to view the series of radiographic images associated with the exam report (step 21). MINDscape formulates a common gateway interface (CGI) query (step 22) using the unique examination accession number provided to it by the RIS. The image series for the unique RIS accession number used in step 22 is retrieved from the Web server and transmitted to the user's browser where a plug-in (or helper program) is used to decompress and display the images (step 23; see Figure 5.3) with the customary array of image manipulation tools (zoom, window/level, mensuration, and so on).

In the sections that follow, we aim to familiarize you with the various standards, technologies, and transactions described in the many steps of the scenario process decomposition. The casual reader may wish to skim or skip over some or all of these sections.

Health Level 7

Health Level 7 (HL7) was founded in 1987 to develop standards for the electronic interchange of clinical, financial, and administrative information among independent healthcare-oriented computer systems, e.g., hospital information systems, clinical laboratory systems, enterprise systems, and pharmacy systems. The current HL7 standard defines a transaction syntax for the transfer of data among the multitude of healthcare information system applications in the various environments in which healthcare is delivered that send or receive medical data. These include patient admissions/registration, discharge or transfer (ADT) data, insurance, billing and payers, orders and results for diagnostic tests, nursing and physician observations, pharmacy orders, and resource/patient scheduling. HL7 is currently developing transactions for exchanging information about problem lists, clinical trial enrollments, patient permissions, voice dictations, advance directives, and physiologic waveforms.

HL7 does not try to assume a particular architecture with respect to the placement of data within applications but is designed to support a central patient care system as well as a more distributed environment where data reside in departmental systems like radiology and laboratory medicine. Message formats prescribed in the HL7 encoding rules consist of data fields that are of variable length and separated by a field separator character. Rules describe how the various data types are encoded within a field and when an individual field may be repeated. The data fields are combined into logical groupings called segments. Each segment begins with a three-character literal value that identifies it within a message (e.g., ORM—general order message). Individual data fields are found in the HL7 message by their position within their associated segments. For more details regarding HL-7 interfaces see Chapter 3, p. 24.

Image Acquisition with Digital Imaging and Communications in Medicine (DICOM)

In 1982, the American College of Radiology (ACR) and the National Electrical Manufacturers Association (NEMA) formed a joint committee to develop a standard for the transfer of medical images between imaging devices and computers. This has evolved into the Digital Imaging and Communications in Medicine (DICOM) standard. The essence of the DICOM standard is that it prescribes a uniform, well-understood set of rules for the communication of digital images. This has been accomplished through defining, as unambiguously as possible, the terms it uses and in defining object-oriented models for medical imaging information. The DICOM standard is extremely adaptable, a planned feature that has led to the adoption of DICOM by other medical specialties that generate images in the course of patient diagnosis and treatment (e.g., cardiology, endoscopy, and ophthalmology).[3]

DICOM Service-Object Pairs

The fundamental functional unit of DICOM is the service-object pair (SOP). Everything implemented in DICOM is based on the use of SOP classes. The elemental units that make up the SOP are information objects and service classes. As DICOM was founded on an object-oriented design philosophy, things such as images, reports, and patients are all objects in DICOM and are termed information objects. The definition of what constitutes an information object in DICOM is called an information object definition (IOD), which is basically a structured list of attributes. An example of a DICOM IOD is that of a CT image (CT image IOD). Once the attributes (e.g., patient identification number) are "filled in," the object then becomes an information object instance.

Another elemental unit of DICOM is the service class. Information objects and the communications links between devices are not sufficient in and of themselves to provide functionality; it is necessary that these devices perform some operation (service) on the information objects. Some of the many DICOM services are Storage, Query/Retrieve, Print, and Modality Worklist Management. Because of the object-oriented nature of DICOM, services are referred to as service classes; a given service may be applied to a variety (or class) of information objects (e.g., Storage Service Class). A distinction is also made based on whether the device acts as a user or provider of a given service.

The service classes and information objects are then combined to form service object pairs (SOPs). The process of DICOM communication involves the exchange of SOP instances through the use of DICOM messages. For example, the transfer and storage of a specific CT image to a DICOM archiving computer represents a CT image storage SOP instance. If the device is accepting the image object for storage (e.g., the DICOM archiving computer), it is termed a Storage Service Class Provider (storage SCP). The device that requests the image to be stored (e.g., the CT scanner) is termed a Storage Service Class User (Storage SCU). Therefore, at a minimum, each digital imaging modality should act as a DICOM Storage SCU for its specific image object (e.g., CT IOD).

DICOM Storage Service Class

Images for PACS can be received directly from the modality in digital format or indirectly through analog film or video digitization.[4] The advantage of direct digital capture is that it affords the radiologist access to the entire original digital data set without truncation of image matrix dimension, spatial resolution, or pixel bit depth. The latter gives the radiologist and or primary care physician full capability in adjusting image window and level settings. There are image quality losses in the process of going from a digital representation to an analog medium and then digitizing the analog medium, but it has proved difficult to quantify their significance. For example, analog video frame grabbing is still used at some institutions to print CT images to laser film printers, and there is little visual loss of information aside from the inability to visualize the full 12-bit data set. Digitization of the laser-printed multislice CT film can, however, cause loss of spatial resolution, loss of contrast resolution, and possibly moiré patterns or other artifacts.

The DICOM standard has become the predominant standard for the communication of medical images, and it allows for the direct digital transfer of images from, say, a CT or MR scanner to a PACS, as discussed previously. The Storage Service Class defines an application-level class of service that facilitates the simple transfer of images between software processes on computers termed application entities (AEs). Two peer DICOM AEs implement an SOP Class of the Storage Service Class with one serving in the SCU role and one serving in the SCP role. Storage SOP Classes are intended to be used in a variety of environments, e.g., for modalities to transfer images to workstations or archives, for archives to transfer images to workstations or back to modalities, for workstations to transfer processed images to archives, and so on.

Acquisition Mechanisms for Non-DICOM Modalities

Film Digitizers

The most common device for analog image acquisition is the film digitizer. Film digitizers convert to digital format the still ubiquitous conventional projection radiographic films captured using screen-film technology or laser-printed multiformat films from digital modalities (e.g., a CT scanner) that don't provide DICOM storage SCU. There are two major competing technologies in the film digitizer marketplace. Laser film digitizers, the past and current gold standard of film digitization, offer superior contrast and spatial resolution, but they are expensive. Current-generation charged-coupled device (CCD) digitizers offer comparable (or greater) spatial resolution than laser film digitizers, but many manufactured systems employing CCDs fall somewhat short on contrast resolution.[5] CCD digitizers are typically smaller, lighter, and less costly than laser-based digitizers. CCD digitizers are also easier to maintain, as there is no rotating or vibrating mirror to adjust periodically. The optical components in a CCD digitizer are also much simpler than those found in laser digitizers.[6]

Ideally, the range of optical densities the film digitizer is capable of capturing should span the entire range encountered clinically. For all applications with the exception of mammography this equates to a dynamic range of $10^{3.5}$ (optical density range 0.0 to 3.5).

Film digitizers vary as to the spatial resolution (usually assumed to be the digitization spot size, typically 200 microns down to 25 microns), the contrast resolution (number of useable bits, typically 8 to 16), whether multiple film sizes are handled, whether the digitization spot size is variable, and whether only single sheets are handled or multiple sheets can be batch loaded using a sheetfeeding mechanism. To adhere to the ACR teleradiology equipment guidelines,[7] a 200-micron digitization element (2.5 line pairs/mm) and a bit depth of at least 10 bits per pixel must be used. For a $14'' \times 17''$ radiographic film, this equates to a digitization matrix of 1780×2160 and a bit depth of 12 bits per pixel, but stored along 16-bit (2-byte) boundaries results in a file size of 7.4 megabytes.

Video Frame Grabbers

If an imaging system has video output signal, such as an ultrasound scanner or fluoroscopic system with a vidicon camera, a video frame grabber can be used to digitize these temporally varying one-dimensional signals into a two-dimensional digital image. One major problem with the use of video is that contrast resolution is curtailed to 8 bits by typically used digital-to-analog converter electronics. This isn't really a problem with ultrasound images, which have a useful data bit depth of only 6 to 8 bits, but it poses problems for modalities like CT and MRI where the ability to adjust the window and level settings of the images is severely compromised and thus useful diagnostic information is lost. It is possible to video frame grab at multiple window and level settings and save them to PACS (exactly as if they were being printed to film with, say, soft tissue, lung, and bone windows for CT). However, this requires additional work on the part of the radiology technologist, more data to be transmitted, and a greater number of images for the radiologist to manage and interpret on the display workstation.

Picture Archiving and Communication Systems (PACS)

At the heart of the digital revolution in the radiology department is PACS. PACS is a complex collection of computing hardware, software, and workflow processes aimed at replacing the hard copy film environment with digital acquisition, transfer, storage, and display of radiographic images (refer to Figure 5.4). The digital acquisition component has already been addressed and usually occurs directly on the acquisition modalities (e.g., CT and MR). A network, typically a local area network or extensions of multiple local area networks between various sites of practice are required for the computers to intercommunicate.[8] Key to the discussion of storage is the PACS database and hierarchical storage management (HSM) systems. These databases are usually relational in nature (though object databases have been used) and utilize structured query language (SQL) to access and manipulate the data. Image display is provided either through the use of dedicated high-resolution grayscale and color monitors or through the use of a Web server and ubiquitous Web-browsing software, which usually require plug-ins or Active X components to provide image decompression and window-level functionality.

Local Area Network

Up until about five years ago, local area networks (LANs) made use of shared, broadcasting approaches to support communication among computers (e.g., shared 10 megabit/sec—Mbps—Ethernet). Since then, switched LANs have been used, and now, 100-Mbps and gigabit (1000 Mbps) switched Ethernet LANs have become commonplace for PACS installations. Ethernet equipment purchased today uses switching and full-duplex operation to provide maximum signaling bandwidth to and from the host computer. It also makes use of the same transport control protocol/Internet protocol (TCP/IP) stack, as does the larger and worldwide Internet.

The core PACS components (e.g., archive, database, and Web server) are usually located in an environmentally controlled and secure computer room. These core components are typically connected to an Ethernet switch with multimode fiber-optic connections that support 1 Gbps (gigabit per second) transfer rates. All other PACS components, either inside or outside the computer room, and scanners are connected through 100-Mbps Ethernet connections using Category 5 unshielded twisted pair (UTP) wiring. The PACS computer room Ethernet switch is connected to other switches and routers in the medical center through redundant gigabit fiber-optic links. The connection from these switches to the PACS workstations and to the physician desktop is through 100-Mbps UTP Ethernet, terminated at a wall jack.

Relational Database and Structured Query Language

In 1969, E. F. Codd developed a relational theory of data, which he proposed as a universal foundation for database systems. His relational model, based on the set mathematics of relations and first-order predicate logic, covers the three aspects of data that any database management system (DBMS) must address: structure, integrity, and manipulation. An informal definition of a relational DBMS is that it represents all information in the database as tables, it supports the three relational operations known as selection, projection and join for specifying exactly what data you want to see, and it uses a single high-level language for structuring, querying, and changing the information in the database.

A set of related tables forms the database. Example tables in the PACS database include STAFF__AND__REFERRING__PHYSICIANS, PROCEDURES, and REFERRING__SERVICE. Each row describes one instantiation of an entity in the table, for example, a specific CT procedure (e.g., "CT Head w/o Contrast") in the PROCEDURES table. Each column describes one characteristic of the entity. Example entities for the PROCEDURE entity include procedure__code, procedure__desc, and modality__code. Each data element in the table can be identified as the intersection of a row (x axis) and column (y axis).

The definition of a relational system (and Codd's rules) requires that a single language (also known as comprehensive data sublanguage) be able to handle all communications with the database. This language is the structured query language (SQL, pronounced "see-quel"). SQL is used for data manipulation (retrieval and modification), data definition, and data administration. That is, every retrieval, definition, or administrative operation is expressed as a SQL statement.

There are two varieties of data manipulation operations—data retrieval and data modification. Retrieval means finding the particular data one wants; modification means adding, removing, or changing the data in a table. Data retrieval operations (or queries) search the database, fetch information that has been requested by the most efficient means possible, and display it. A generic SQL query on a table might look like "select SELECT__ATTRIBUTES from TABLE__LIST where SEARCH CONDITIONS." For example, using the PATIENT__DESCRIPTION table for a query, select PATIENT__ID, DATE__OF__BIRTH, SEX from PATIENT__DESCRIPTION where SEX = "M" would result in a SQL return (data output) something like Table 5.1.

Archive: Hierarchical Storage Management Systems

Hierarchical storage management (HSM) systems usually consist of a hierarchy of digital storage media selected to fit speed/capacity/media cost criterion. Most have a front-end, short-term archiving unit with many gigabytes of fast magnetic discs (RAID level 5) that can stream requested images to display stations at a rate of around 80 Mbps and act as a buffer for the slower, long-term archiving units using optical disc and/or magnetic tape libraries. HSM systems also manage the migration of images and related data that have not been accessed for a period of

TABLE 5.1 A data output table resulting from the structured query select PATIENT_ID, DATE_OF_BIRTH, SEX from PATIENT_DESCRIPTION where SEX = "M".

PATIENT_ID	DATE_OF_BIRTH	SEX
U0439675	730530	M
U0555767	510704	M
•	•	•
•	•	•
•	•	•
U9959675	280421	M

time to the longer-term archive media, manage the migration of long-term exam images (selected comparison exams) to the short-term RAID when either scheduled (prefetch) or requested on demand (ad hoc), and proactively interrogate long-term media for reliability, rewriting this data to new media if it appears that a specific unit of media is failing.

The main limitations for the quick retrieval required for on-demand de-archiving of exam images from the long-term archive are that optical discs, although a random access medium (access times on the order of 25 msec), have slow data transfer rates (maximum 5 megabytes/second—MBps) and are relatively expensive ($13/gigabyte—GB—uncompressed). Digital magnetic tape, on the other hand, is relatively inexpensive ($3.5/GB) and has phenomenal data transfer rates (upward of 20 MBps), but as a sequential access medium, tape has mean file access times on the order of 10 seconds.

Smaller files (e.g., a PA and lateral chest exam—15 MB) favor optical disc storage. Large files, like CT and MR examinations with hundreds of images or those found outside radiology (e.g., cine fluorography and echo cardiology) involving long segments of video frames, favor storage on magnetic tape. For example, the average CT examination at our institution with high-speed, multiplanar image acquisition is around 200 MB. If we were to access a CT exam from optical disc it would take at least 40 seconds (25 msec access time + 40 sec transfer time), whereas from digital magnetic tape, it takes approximately 20 seconds (10 sec access time + 10 sec reading time). Retrieving a PA and lateral chest exam would require 3 seconds for optical disc and 10 seconds for magnetic tape. This estimate discounts any time required for the robotics to find the media in the archive library and insert them into an available reader, which is assumed to be the same for both media (about 10 sec).

Web Server

A Web server responds to universal resource locator (URL) requests generated by a user's Web browser through services like the Hypertext Transfer Protocol (HTTP) by returning the solicited Hypertext Markup Language (HTML) document, which is then displayed in the Web browser window after parsing the

HTML document. If one wants more than simple static pages returned, then the URL can contain a Common Gateway Interface (CGI) query. The CGI is the standard by which external programs (often called gateways or gateway programs) can interface with an HTTP (Web) server. The CGI program (or script) can be designed to handle an information request to a database, take the results and assemble an HTML document from them and return this document to the user's Web browser. Thus CGI programs act as gateways between the HTTP server and databases or between the server and local programs or document generators.

An efficient mechanism for image display through MINDscape is for the referring or primary care physician to find the patient list of radiological examinations (refer to Figure 5.1) they are interested in and select a hyperlink button that then invokes the PACS Web server to present images from that specific examination.[9] This is performed using a CGI query to the PACS Web server that includes the RIS accession number for that specific radiology exam report. An example of this CGI query might be "https://pacs.washington.edu/study__list.cgi?accno=754028&patid=U6999999&namelast=TESTMCIS&namefirst=PTIGNORE". Please note that "https" denotes the secure version of HTTP, as discussed later. As most of the DICOM images transferred from the imaging modalities have the RIS accession number embedded in the associated DICOM header data attribute field (tag number = 0008,0050), the PACS Web server can find the relevant examination image series and display it directly to the user's browser (refer to Figure 5.4). No navigation through the PACS Web server database is required, and the large volumes of images (4–8 terabytes—TB) per year for a major teaching institution are not duplicated strictly within the EMR database. Typically, an appropriately sized Web server or cluster of Web servers can service hundreds of concurrent users.

Image Display

The images from a PACS are usually displayed in either of two methods. The first is through the use of dedicated high-resolution grayscale (CT, MR, digital and computed radiography, and digital fluoroscopy) and color monitors (ultrasound, nuclear medicine, and PET). These workstations usually cost tens of thousands of dollars. The second method is through the use of a Web server and ubiquitous and free Web-browsing software, which usually requires plug-ins (e.g., Netscape Navigator) or Active X (e.g., Microsoft Internet Explorer) components to provide image decompression and window-level functionality.

Dedicated PACS display workstations are usually commercial off-the-shelf PCs using the NT operating system. Additional memory (up to 1 GB) may be added in addition to special display cards with multiple frame buffers (e.g., 2048 by 2560 by 16 bits) for use with two or four high-fidelity, high-resolution display monitors. If color display is used, then a single high-performance display card of sufficient resolution (e.g., 1600 by 1200 by 24 bits—"true color") is used to drive one or two monitors. Basic image-manipulation tools include intensity transformation tables (automatic preset window/level, manual window/level control, and image invert), image enlargement and translation (zoom and roam), and mensuration (calibrated distances and calculated angle measurements). In addition, the ability to add and hide graphic overlays (scanner information, manually entered text annotations, arrows, or regions of interest) and rotation capabilities are important.

To display the images from the Web server in a timely manner over most Internet connection speeds (256–1024 kbps for DSL and cable modem), compression is often used. Unless a ubiquitous compression algorithm programmed into the native Web browser software (e.g., lossy 8-bit JPEG compression), a plug-in or Active X component must be utilized for image decompression (e.g., wavelet compression). The compression ratio of any specific image is a dynamic function of the modality type, and the inherent detail and contrast of each image. In addition, the plug-in allows manipulation of the full 12-bit and 16-bit contrast resolution of CT and MR images, respectively. The plug-in or Active X component also performs the following image-manipulation functions: window/level, flip, invert, sort, rotate, zoom, cine-loop, and save as lossy JPEG. The required plug-in or Active X component is usually stored on the Web server itself for easy installation.

Image Compression

Medical image data sets are relatively large and image compression plays a valuable role. A computed radiograph (CR) of 1760 by 2140 pixels and a 10-bit pixel depth requires 7.5 megabytes of digital storage. A CT examination consisting of 200 images requires 100 megabytes. Obviously, image compression must be used judiciously as it generally trades image quality for compression ratio. This is especially important when low-bandwidth connectivity (e.g., a 33.6 kbps modem) is used. With lossless compression the original images can be exactly reconstituted (bit for bit), so there is no degradation in image quality unless there is an error in the transfer of the image data (this is usually corrected by the network protocol stack. Lossy compression techniques cause a varying amount of degradation in image quality, depending on image feature characteristics and the degree of compression.

Lossless compression schemes typically permit compression ratios (the numerator is the number of bytes required for storage of the original image and the denominator is the number of bytes required for storage of the compressed image) of between 2:1 and 4:1 reduction in the number of bytes required to represent an image. Techniques that claim compression ratios exceeding 4:1 are almost certainly lossy. Vendors euphemistically term this "visually" lossless (*caveat emptor*). Compression ratios closer to 10:1 or 20:1 are required to have a significant practical and economic impact. Although the medical community did not readily embrace the concept of lossy data compression initially, there is sufficient evidence that such schemes can be implemented without compromising the diagnostic content of images.[10,11,12]

Even though compression may cause a loss of image quality, radiographs compressed by as much as 10:1 to 20:1 and CT and MR images compressed by 5:1 to 8:1 are in most cases acceptable for clinical review. In the current healthcare environment, which stresses cost effectiveness, a slight reduction in image quality may be offset by financial considerations such as increased capacity of the image storage media and reduced image network transfer and transmission times. Compression may be performed through either software or special hardware. There is a trade-off between the speed of compression and decompression and the monetary cost of the compression mechanism. Software-based compression methods are usually slower than special hardware compression boards but cost much less than the hardware solutions and are typically more flexible.

Security

As our society relies more and more on the Internet to communicate and do business, healthcare is also taking advantage of the "information superhighway." As healthcare information, including medical image transmission, shifts further and further from private networks and intranets to the Internet, enhanced security of individually identifiable patient information becomes a prime concern [Baur 1997].

HIPAA and HCFA Requirements

A national debate about how and how much to protect the privacy of personal health data entered and stored in computers and transferred electronically has simmered for approximately 25 years without resolution. The Health Insurance Portability and Accountability Act of 1996 (HIPAA) [NRC 1997] has forced resolution and compromise quickly. The health privacy rules in the HIPAA legislation are a requisite to implementing the administrative simplification provisions of HIPAA that mandate use of a uniform, electronic data set for financial and administrative transactions and a unique identifier for every participant in the health system.

Along with this, the Health Care Financing Administration (HCFA) had until October 1998 a long-standing policy of banning the Internet for the communication of individually identifiable patient information. HCFA has come to recognize that its ban on the use of the Internet is inconsistent with technology trends, economics, and new federal policies and rules, not the least of which are the forthcoming HIPAA-mandated security regulations. HCFA drafted a new policy in October 1998 that provides HCFA contractors with guidelines for the appropriate use of the Internet. HCFA policies apply officially only to the information protected under the Privacy Act of 1974, which is a mandate on federal agencies. In the healthcare context, this act protects information about patients covered under Medicare, Medicaid, and federal child insurance programs. However, the HIPAA legislation will almost assuredly increase the scope of this policy to apply to all patient information.

As more and more PACS move toward Web server operation over the Internet from the point-to-point dial-up modem model, the HCFA policy guidelines and HIPAA legislation will have great impact on future teleradiology transactions. It will be permissible to use the Internet for transmission of individually identifiable patient information or other sensitive healthcare data as long as an acceptable method of encryption is utilized to provide confidentiality and integrity of the data. Also required is the employment of authentication or identification procedures to assure that both the sender and the recipient of the data are known to each other and are authorized to receive such information. Neither the HCFA policy nor HIPAA legislation spells out the exact mechanisms to be used for these functions, as encryption and authentication technologies are moving targets.

Authentication

Authentication is the process of identifying an individual, usually by a username and password but extending now into biometric (fingerprint and retinal) identification as well as "smart cards." A smart card is a small device the size of a credit card that displays a constantly changing user ID code. A user first enters a password into the computer and then the card displays a user ID that can be used authentication. Typically, the user IDs change every 1 to 5 minutes. In security systems, authentication is distinct from authorization, which is the process of giving individuals access to system functions based on their identity. Authentication merely ensures that the individual is who he or she claims to be; it says nothing about the access rights of the individual.

A certificate authority (CA) is a trusted third-party organization or company that issues digital certificates used to create digital signatures and public–private key pairs. The role of the CA in this process is to guarantee that the individual granted the unique certificate is, in fact, who they claim to be. Usually, this means that the CA has an arrangement with a financial institution, such as a credit card company, that provides it with information to confirm an individual's claimed identity. Certificate authorities are a critical component in authentication security on the Web because they guarantee that the two parties exchanging information are really who they claim to be. Every secure sockets layer (SSL) server must have an SSL server certificate. When a Web browser connects to a Web server using the SSL protocol, the server sends the browser its public key in an X.509 certificate.

Encryption

Encryption is the transformation of data to conceal its information content, prevent undetected modification, and/or prevent its unauthorized use. Encryption uses a single or multiple keys. Key management is then required when encryption is used. There are two main types of encryption: asymmetric encryption (also called public key encryption) and symmetric encryption (also called private key encryption). Encryption may use hardware or software. Currently, most systems employing encryption use software. Two methods are secure sockets layer (SSL) and secure MIME (S/MIME).

SSL is a protocol developed for transmitting private documents via the Internet. SSL works by using a private key to encrypt data that is transferred over the SSL connection. SSL is a protocol to authenticate server to client and (potentially) client to server, to establish a "session," and to negotiate parameters for the encryption of messages exchanged during a session. These parameters include a shared "symmetric" encryption key and chosen encryption algorithm. SSL does not require any particular choice of these parameters. Both the Netscape Navigator and Internet Explorer browsers support SSL, and many Web sites use the protocol to obtain confidential user information. By convention, Web pages that require an SSL connection start with https: rather than http:. SSL comes in multiple strengths using various length (e.g., 40, 56, 128, and 168 bits) encryption keys. SSL using an encryption key greater than 40 bits is termed "strong" encryption. Using "default" SSL configurations in browsers and servers probably results in no client authentication and 40-bit encryption.

MIME (multipurpose Internet mail extensions) is a specification for formatting non-ASCII messages so that they can be sent over the Internet. S/MIME is a protocol for the cryptographic enveloping of MIME messages. Because e-mail is asynchronous, the sender determines algorithm/key length prior to sending the S/MIME message. S/MIME itself does not determine key length; it determines merely how to securely exchange keys and algorithm information. S/MIME implementations usually support a number of algorithms, but the standard requires support for only relatively weak algorithms (due to the federal export restriction and patent concerns). The sender choosing relatively strong encryption may find some recipients unable to decipher the message, while relatively insecure messages will routinely be received and decrypted. For example, Netscape's domestic S/MIME implementation's default configuration calls for 168 bits (triple DES (data encryption standard)).

Virtual Private Networks

A virtual private network (VPN) allows one to connect from one's office or home or on the road to an enterprise's central networks using the Internet to securely transmit private data. VPNs eliminate the expense of special leased line connections and long-distance dial-up. VPNs secure private network traffic by encrypting the data stream using a variety of standard algorithms (e.g., triple DES), authenticating incoming connections to assure the integrity of the source, and managing encryption key distribution and exchange for access control to data. Using these security measures, VPN devices construct virtual point-to-point tunnels through the Internet between remote users and the central network. When an authorized user logs off, the connection simply collapses.

The medical center would support one or multiple VPN servers on subnetworks. These devices can handle hundreds of simultaneous connections. The client computer connecting to the VPN server over the Internet makes use of a program (typically freely distributed by the server vendor) to connect with the server's IP using a password and/or digital certificates. Once the user is logged into the VPN server account, the user can access systems on the subnetworks that are specified in the account authorization list. The client software automatically forwards all Ethernet packets bound for those subnetworks through the client encryption algorithm and to the VPN server, which decrypts the packets and injects them onto the medical center network. Packets bound for other Internet entities (e.g., Yahoo) are unmolested. Images transmitted from the medical center are encrypted by the VPN server, transmitted across the Internet to the client computer's program, and decrypted for use or manipulation. Any Internet service provider (ISP) connection to the Internet—e.g., cable modem, digital subscriber line (DSL), satellite, leased line, or simple dial-up modem connections—can access the VPN server.

References

1. Dwyer SJ. Imaging system architectures for picture archiving and communication systems. *Radiol Clin North Am* 34:495–503; 1996.
2. Huang HK. *PACS: Picture Archiving and Communication Systems in Biomedical Imaging.* New York: VCH; 1996.
3. Bidgood WD, Horii SC. Modular extension of the ACR-NEMA DICOM standard to support new diagnostic imaging modalities and services. *J Digit Imaging* 1996;9:67–77.
4. Horii SC. Image acquisiton: sites, technologies, and approaches. *Radiol Clin North Am* 1996;34:469–94.
5. Hangiandreou NJ, O'Connor TJ, Felmlee JP. An evaluation of the signal and noise characteristics of four CCD-based film digitizers. *Med Phys* 1998;25: 2020–26.
6. Forsberg DA. Quality assurance in teleradiology. *Telemed J* 1995;1:107–14.
7. Stewart BK. *Teleradiology.* 1999 AAPM Summer School on Digital Radiology, Sonoma State University, CA. Medical Physics Publishing, Madison, WI, 1999, pp. 403–32.
8. Stewart BK. *Networks, Pipes and Connectivity.* 1999 AAPM Summer School on Digital Radiology, Sonoma State University, CA. Medical Physics Publishing, Madison, WI, 1999, pp. 259–86.
9. Stewart BK, Langer SG, Martin KP. Integration of multiple DICOM Web-servers into an enterprise-wide Web-based electronic medical record. *Proc SPIE* 1999;3662:52–59.
10. Aberle DR, Gleeson F, Sayre JW, et al. The effect of irreversible image compression on diagnostic accuracy in thoracic imaging. *Invest Radio 1* 1993;28: 398–403.
11. Bolle SR, Sund T, Stormer J. Receiver operating characteristic study of image preprocessing for teleradiology and digital workstations. *J Digit Imaging* 1997;10:152–57.
12. Good WF, Maitz GS, Gur D. Joint photographic experts group (JPEG) compatible data compression of mammograms. *J Digital Imaging* 1994;7:123–32.

6
Evidence-Based Medicine

John P. Geyman, M.D. and Fredric M. Wolf, Ph.D.

Scenario 1

A 59-year-old man presents to your office with a 4 week history of intermittent substernal chest discomfort with exertion, without radiation and relieved by rest. Each of several episodes lasted no more than 5 minutes. He has been in good general health, had no history of prior chest pain, hypertension, diabetes, or serious illness. He is a nonsmoker and takes no medications. Family history reveals that his father died at age 73, probably of myocardial infarction.

Physical examination reveals a middle-aged man in no distress with blood pressure 138/88, pulse 80 and regular, respirations 20 per minute, and afebrile. Weight is 200 pounds, height 70 inches. Neck veins are flat, heart NSR without murmurs, lungs clear P & A, abdomen without organomegaly, and extremities without edema. The remainder of the physical examination is within normal limits.

Initial laboratory studies include normal CBC and electrolyte panel. Creatinine is 1.2 mg/dL. Resting ECG is normal, and a stress ECG shows 2-mm ST-segment depression in three leads without blood pressure drop or arrhythmia.

A diagnosis of stable angina pectoris is made; appropriate explanation, counseling, and reassurance are given to the patient; he is started on a diet and exercise program; he is given a prescription for sublingual nitroglycerine. The physician is aware that additional treatment with a long-acting nitrate, beta blocker, or calcium channel blocker might also be helpful. He looks up this issue in a recent textbook, but is still undecided as to the most effective and safe line of therapy.

This scenario provides a good example of how evidence-based approaches can be useful in everyday practice and actually answer a common clinical question at the point of care. A few years ago, this physician had to rely on textbooks (often outdated even when just published), his own training and clinical experience, and the advice of consultants who often differed among themselves because of individual global "expert" judgments. The physician had no way of quickly comparing the efficacy, side effects, and comparative outcomes of the three lines of therapy for this patient.

Today, however, the physician with some background and interest in evidence-based medicine can answer these kinds of questions within a few minutes through a targeted search of an electronic resource that he has bookmarked on his office and/or home computer. He consults infoPOEMs, a Web site developed by an editorial group for *The Journal of Family Practice,* and finds an index of over 300 articles that have been rigorously reviewed and abstracted on the basis of three criteria: (1) each article addresses a clinical question encountered by a typical family physician at least once every 6 months; (2) each article measures patient-oriented outcomes important to patients, such as mortality, morbidity, and quality of life; (3) each article reports results that will require a change of practice. The physician scrolls through the index, finds that his question has been addressed, and prints out the abstract. He finds a recent meta-analysis published in *JAMA* in 1999 that analyzed 90 studies on the treatment of angina with nitrate, beta blocker, and calcium channel blocker.[1] Comparative effectiveness of the three different therapies were evaluated in terms of number of angina episodes per week, number of nitroglycerine tablets used per week, total exercise time, and time to 1-mm ST-segment depression during exercise. Tolerability was assessed by recording the rates of patient withdrawal due to adverse events (death or cardiac or noncardiac symptoms).

The meta-analysis yielded good evidence that beta blockers are more effective and better tolerated than calcium channel blockers and should be first-line drugs for treating stable angina. Long-acting nitrates were found to be associated with an increase in *prn* use of sublingual nitroglycerine and are recommended only as second-line agents. Thus, in this instance, the physician is able to answer his question and proceed with a well-grounded treatment plan for this patient after only a brief computer search.

Genesis of Evidence-Based Medicine

Various major trends in healthcare over the last 15 to 20 years have brought increased scrutiny to how clinical decisions are made. These trends have favored a climate for the development of evidence-based approaches for the care of both individuals and populations. Extreme geographic variations in the care of some medical conditions can clearly not be justified in terms of credible variations in the global judgment of experts. Wennberg's work led the way in these studies, finding, for example, 20-fold differences in utilization rates for carotid endarterectomy in 16 large communities in four states.[2] Many other studies of this kind have followed and raised serious questions about the integrity of clinical decision-making processes that can allow such large variations in care. More recently, increasing numbers of clinical guidelines have been produced by various groups, some within the same specialty, others crossing specialty lines and representing various agencies. Many have been promulgated on the basis of global subjective judgments by "experts," not by systematic and rigorous evaluation of all available evidence. As more pervasive examples of the gap between evidence and clinical practice have come to light, and as the need for cost containment has become more apparent in an era of increasingly obvious limits, concepts of evidence-based medicine have found fertile ground for growth. In an environment of increasing information overload, this development has been greatly accelerated

TABLE 6.1 Paradigm shift.

Former paradigm (global expert judgment)	NEW paradigm (evidence-based medicine)
1. Unsystematic observations from clinical experience are valid ways to practice.	1. Clinical experience alone, while essential, does not provide a sufficient guide and is enhanced by systematic observations that are unbiased and reproducible; clinical experience of individual clinicians and groups can be misleading.
2. Study of basic mechanisms of disease and pathophysiology provide acceptable guidance for practice.	
3. Traditional medical education (with emphasis on global judgment by "experts") and common sense allow the clinician to effectively evaluate new tests and therapies.	2. Rationales for diagnosis and treatment derived from the study and understanding of basic mechanisms of disease may be inaccurate and are not sufficient to guide clinical practice.
4. Content expertise and clinical experience provide a sufficient base for valid guidelines for clinical practice.	3. Understanding and applying accepted rules of evidence is necessary to correctly interpret the medical literature concerning causation, natural history, prognosis, diagnostic tests, and treatment options.

Source: Adapted from Evidence-Based Working Group, Evidence-based medicine: A new approach to teaching the practice of medicine, *JAMA* 1992;268:2420–5. Used with permission.

by advances in medical informatics and creation of increasingly useful clinical electronic databases. (see Chapter 8, Knowledge Resources)

Rooted in clinical epidemiology, evidence-based medicine searches out relevant evidence on clinical questions through critical assessment of clinical epidemiologic studies, meta-analysis of randomized clinical trials, decision analysis, and cost-effectiveness analysis. Clinical practice guidelines and pathways of care can thereby be founded on best evidence. Further, process and outcome measures can be identified that can become useful in monitoring quality of care.

The Evidence-Based Medicine Working Group in 1992 compared evidence-based medicine with the global expert judgment approach so entrenched in traditional medical education. The differences are of such magnitude that evidence-based medicine has become viewed as sufficiently different to qualify as a paradigm shift, as conceived by Thomas Kuhn.[3,4] (Table 6.1)

Four basic steps are inherent in the process of evidence-based medicine:[5]

1. Select specific clinical questions from the patient's problem(s).
2. Search the literature or databases for relevant clinical information.
3. Appraise the evidence for validity and usefulness to the patient and practice.
4. Implement useful findings in everyday practice.

Sackett and his colleagues defined evidence-based medicine as the "conscientious, explicit and judicious use of current best evidence in making decisions about the care of individual patients."[6] Since evidence is not available on many clinical questions in everyday practice, the practice of evidence-based medicine

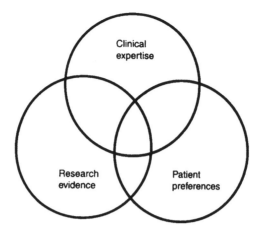

FIGURE 6.1. Basic model for evidence-based clinical decisions as conceived by Haynes and his colleagues.

requires the integration, patient by patient, of the physician's clinical experience and judgment with the best available external evidence. Further, it requires tailoring of best evidence to the particular preferences and needs of the patient or family in a process of informed partnership decision making. Figure 6.1 illustrates the basic model for evidence-based clinical decisions as conceived by Haynes and his colleagues.[7]

Evidence-Based Medicine and Information Mastery

It has been apparent from the beginning of clinicians' attempts to implement evidence-based concepts that the process must be time-efficient and rewarding in terms of answering clinical questions at the point of care. Faced with increasing administrative and emotional burdens of practice, clinicians must be able to quickly find relevant evidence on their questions. Slawson and his colleagues have conceptualized this situation in terms of a usefulness equation:[8]

$$\text{Usefulness} = \frac{\text{relevance} \times \text{validity}}{\text{work}}$$

There are two major sources of evidence, primary and secondary. Primary evidence is found in original bibliographic citations, as found, for example, in Medline, PubMed or other databases. Secondary sources include structured reviews, often in abstract form, by clinicians expert in critical appraisal of primary citations. The use of secondary sources speeds up the search process by busy clinicians, since the primary sources have already been screened for clinical relevance and scientific rigor. Slawson, Shaughnessy, and Bennett have provided a time-

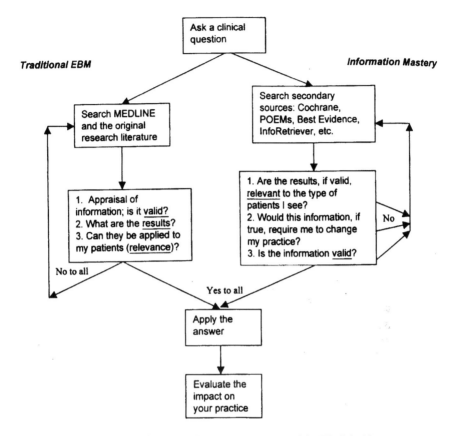

FIGURE 6.2. Model of the direct search process as proposed by Ebell in his paper on answering clinical questions at the point of care. Used with permission by JABFP, 1999; 12:3.

efficient approach to practicing evidence-based medicine by shortcutting the process through information mastery.[8,9] This more direct search process is well illustrated in Figure 6.2, as proposed by Ebell in his important paper on answering clinical questions at the point of care.[10]

Present Status of Evidence-Based Medicine

The last 10 years have seen a steadily growing interest in the application of evidence-based principles to clinical practice. Each year more books, journals, articles, and clinically relevant electronic databases appear. Evidence-based approaches are infiltrating predoctoral and graduate medical education, and a growing number of CME courses are presenting evidence-based content. The Agency for Health Care Policy and Research, now the Agency for Health Care Research and Quality (AHRQ), established 12 evidence-based practice centers in 1997, each charged with the study and assessment of assigned clinical areas. Topics currently under study and review include asthma, otitis media, gastroesophageal reflux disease, and osteoporosis, all common conditions in everyday clinical practice. The AHRQ in collaboration with the American Medical Association and the American Association of Health Plans has also created the National Guideline Clearinghouse in an effort to bring scientific rigor to the assessment and dissemination of clinical practice guidelines.

Today, there are many useful print references available to interested clinicians on evidence-based medicine, as well as user-friendly electronic databases to answer clinical questions. Table 6.2 displays some important resources in evidence-based medicine in both print and electronic categories.

Secondary databases that have already synthesized the primary research literature are increasingly thought to be more efficient and effective in identifying relevant evidence for use in clinical settings.[11] These secondary sources include CAT-banks of critically appraised topics, the Best Evidence CD that contains full-text articles from the *ACP Journal Club* and the journal *Evidence-Based Medicine,* POEM (Patient-Oriented Evidence That Matters, in contrast to DOE, Disease-Oriented Evidence), the Cochrane Library, which includes the Cochrane Database of Systematic Reviews (CDSR), and the Database of Abstracts of Reviews of Effectiveness (DARE) of non-Cochrane produced systematic reviews. The classic approach in evidence-based teaching is to advocate that students, residents, and practicing physicians search for evidence in primary database resources like Medline, EMBASE, and PsycINFO that cite primary research studies. However, this is a slow process not well suited to answering questions within the time pressures of busy clinical practice. Much more efficiency can be gained by searching secondary databases that contain critical appraisals and/or syntheses (e.g., meta-analyses, systematic reviews) of the primary research literature on specific topics. These secondary resources offer the advantage of presenting critical reviews of the research reported in primary studies, often with comments on practical relevance and applicability. Examples of these types of resources include Best Evidence, the Cochrane Database of Systematic Reviews, and POEMs. There are even search engines available that might be thought of as tertiary resources in that one search will identify relevant articles listed in multiple secondary databases.[11] Examples of this type of resource are the Internet-based TRIP (Translating Research into Practice) and the hand-held or desktop-based InfoRetriever,' both of which provide the ability to search multiple secondary and/or primary databases at one time without having to repeat the same search over again within each individual database. For example, TRIP provides a simple search mechanism for an "amalgamation of 26 databases of hyperlinks from 'evidence-based' sites around the world."[12] The Cochrane Library could also be viewed as a tertiary database in that one search yields hits in multiple databases.

Scenarios 2 and 3 illustrate some clinical applications of evidence-based principles in everyday practice. Scenario 2 illustrates a common screening issue that comes up frequently with individual patients and also requires a population-based perspective in determining screening protocols within a group practice.

TABLE 6.2 Resources for evidence-based medicine.

Books

1. Eddy D. *Clinical decision making: From theory to practice: A collection of essays from JAMA.* Boston: Jones & Bartlett, 1966.
2. Geyman JP, Deyo RA, Ramsey SD, editors. *Evidence-based clinical practice: Concepts and approaches.* Woburn, MA: Butterworth-Heinemann, 2000.
3. Pareras LG. *Medicine and the Internet: Reference guide.* Philadelphia, Lippincott-Raven, 1996.
4. Sackett DL, Haynes RB, Tugwell P. *Clinical epidemiology: A basic science for clinical medicine,* 2nd ed. Philadelphia, Lippincott-Raven, 1991.
5. Sackett DL, Richardson WS, Rosenberg W, Haynes RB. *Evidence-based medicine: How to practice and teach EBM,* 2nd ed. New York: Churchill Livingstone, 2000.
6. Greenhalgh T. How to Read a Paper: The Basics of Evidence Based Medicine, 2nd edition, London, BMJ Books, 2000.
7. Egger M, Smith GD, Altman D (Editors). Systematic Reviews in Health Care: Meta-Analysis in Context, 2nd edition, London, BMJ Books, 2001.

Articles

1. Bennett JW, Glazious P. Evidence-based practice: What does it really mean? *Dis Manage Health Outcomes* 1997;1:277–85.
2. Ebell MH, Barry HC, Slawson DC, Shaughnessy AF. Finding POEMs in the medical literature. *J Fam Pract* 1999;48:350–5.
3. Evidence-Based Medicine Working Group. A new approach to teaching the practice of medicine. *JAMA* 1992;268:2420–5.
4. Fletcher RH, Fletcher SW. Evidence-based approach to the medical literature. *J Gen Intern Med* 1997;12(Suppl 2)S5–S14.
5. Graber MA, Bergus GR, York C. Using the World Wide Web to answer clinical questions: How efficient are different methods of information retrieval? *J Fam Pract* 1999;48:520–4.
6. Shaughnessy AF, Slawson DC. Getting the most from review articles: A guide for readers and writers. *Am Fam Physician* 1997;55:2155–60.
7. Slawson DC, Shaughnessy AF, Bennett JH. Becoming a medical information master: Feeling good about not knowing everything. *J Fam Pract* 1994;38:505–13.
8. Rosenberg W, Donald A. Evidence-based medicine: An approach to clinical problem-solving. *BMJ* 1995;310:1122–6.
9. Chesanow N. Put a computer in your pocket. *Med Econ* 2000;(October 23):76–8.
10. Chesanow N. Know your needs, pick a device to fit. *Med Econ* 2000;(October 23):81–104.
11. Ebell MH, Frame F. What can technology do to, and for, family practice? *Fam Med* 2001; (in press).
12. Scherger JE. E-mail enhanced relationships: Getting back to basics. *Hippocrates* 1999;(November):7–8.
13. Kassirer JP. Patients, physicians, and the Internet. *Health Aff* (Millwood) 2000;19(6):115–23.

Electronic

1. Best Evidence (http://www.acponline.org/catalogue/cb/best_evidence.htm)
2. InPOEMs (http://www.infopoems.com)
3. PubMed http://www.ncbi.nlm.nih.gov/PubMed
4. Agency for Healthcare Research and Quality (http://www.ahcpr.gov.80/)
5. National Guideline Clearinghouse http://www.guidelines.gov/
6. Health Services/Technology Assessment Text (HSTAT) (http://text.nlm.nih.gov.HSTAT)
7. Bandolier (www.jr2.ox.ac.uK:80/Bandolier)
8. Center for Evidence-Based Medicine (CEBM) (cebm.jr2.ox.ac.uK)
9. Cochrane Collaboration (hiru.mcmaster.ca/COCHRANE
10. Physicians/Online (POL) www.po.com
11. TRIP (Translating Research Into Practice) homepage. http://www.tripdatabase.com/
12. SumSearch homepage (http://sumsearch.uthscsa.edu/searchform5.htm)

Scenario 2

There have been recent differences of opinion and controversy about the effectiveness of a breast screening program for women. As the primary care physician for a 54-year-old healthy woman who asks you for your opinion of the evidence for and against screening, you decide to go to the literature to review the evidence with her. When you conduct a PubMed search of MEDLINE, you discover an article by Tabar and colleagues entitled "Reduction in mortality from breast cancer after mass screening with mammography," which was published in the *Lancet* in 1985.[12] You remember having heard in a continuing medical education course that this is a report of the original Scandinavian multinational randomized trial designed to examine the effectiveness of mammography screening in reducing breast cancer–specific deaths. The abstract indicates that there was a "31% reduction in mortality from breast cancer . . . after seven years of follow-up" for women aged 40 to 74.[13] In looking at the text of the article, you were able to find data for women 50 years and older that indicated that 71 of 58,148 women who had been randomly assigned to the mammography group in comparison to 76 of 41,104 women in the control group had died of breast cancer–specific disease over the seven-year period.

You remember from your statistics and epidemiology training that there are various ways of estimating the effectiveness of the intervention. These effect-size measures include estimates of (1) relative risk reduction, (2) risk difference, (3) reduction in odds of dying, (4) comparison of survival rates, and (5) number of patients needed to treat (or screen) to prevent one adverse event (death, in this example). When you calculate the estimates based on the results of the Tabar et al. study you find the following: The results for women over 50 years old indicate that with mammography, (1) the rate of death was reduced by 34%, (2) there was an absolute reduction in deaths from breast cancer of 0.06%, (3) the rate of patient survival from breast cancer increased from 99.82% to 99.88%, (4) for every 1,588 women who were screened, one breast cancer–specific death was prevented (this is the number needed to treat/screen), and (5) screening reduced the odds of breast cancer–specific death by 34%. You wonder what is the best way to represent and discuss these findings and estimates with your patient.

The various ways in which the results are presented in Scenario 2 are typical of how the results of research studies are reported in professional medical journals and subsequently quoted in the popular press. The glossary of terms provides more formal definitions of each of the five measures of effectiveness, along with the calculations for each based on the Scenario 2 example.

How findings like these are interpreted are critical when physicians, patients, healthcare planners, and policy makers make healthcare decisions. What may not be transparent to people is that each of the five results for each case are really alternative representations of the same research findings and are derived from exactly the same underlying data. This implies that your preference for each intervention, therapeutic or screening, should be identical regardless of how the information is presented. Results of studies using problems like these suggest very clearly that this is not the case, that how information is framed does indeed affect the decisions people make, and that preference reversals do indeed take place when the same evidence is presented in different ways.[14-17] These studies suggest that people are significantly more supportive of using the intervention when outcomes are expressed in terms of relative risk reduction, less supportive when outcomes are expressed as the absolute risk difference or the number of patients needed to treat (or screen) to prevent one patient from experiencing an adverse event (NNT). While each representation of the evidence is "correct," it might be argued that full disclosure would require that all five representations be provided for the most informed decision making to occur.

Scenario 3 illustrates another common clinical question, this time dealing with therapeutic options.

Scenario 3

A 75-year-old woman presents to your office, in the company of her daughter, with gradually increasing memory lapses and some behavioral changes observed by her family. Last week she became lost while driving home after a shopping trip. Her daughter states that her mother has become disorganized in housework and easily confused by financial matters and bookkeeping. The patient has been in good general health over the years, takes no medications, denies alcohol use, and gives no history of headaches, falls, or problems with balance. Her mother lived to the age of 85 and was in a nursing home for her last 6 years, probably with dementia.

Physical examination is within normal limits, including blood pressure of 135/85, pulse 80 with normal sinus rhythm, and normal neurological examination. The patient does not appear to be depressed and responds appropriately to most questions. She seems to lack confidence, however, relying on her daughter for some answers. Her score on the Mini-Mental Status Examination (MMSE) is 24 out of 30 possible points.

Laboratory studies include normal complete blood count, electrolyte panel, TSH, B12 and folate levels, and ECG. A CT scan shows mild-diffuse cortical atrophy and questionable atrophy of the hippocampus.

A clinical diagnosis of early Alzheimer's dementia is made. A neurologist is consulted, who concurs with this diagnosis and suggests that Donepezil may be useful, at least as a holding action. You would like to find out the latest on the efficacy and outcomes of this drug and decide to apply your recent interest in evidence-based medicine in this effort. You visit your bookmarked Web site for the Cochrane Library and are pleased to find a recent abstract addressing this question.

With your new knowledge that Donepezil has produced modest improvements in some patients like yours in both cognitive function and global clinical state, as assessed by their physicians, you discuss this treatment option with the patient and her family. A decision is made to try Donepezil at a 5 mg/day dose for 12 to 24 weeks, and arrangements are made for regular follow-up.

Despite the importance of evidence-based medicine, as hailed by its proponents, the term continues to generate considerable debate. Many clinicians and
medical educators have reacted negatively, some claiming that "that's what we've
always done" and persisting with the global expert judgment patterns of teaching
and practice. Others decry the missionary zeal of some of the proponents of
evidence-based medicine, fearing that clinical experience and judgment will be
replaced by "cookbook medicine." As with many shifts in schools of thought, the
"truth" is probably somewhere between these perceptions.

Moving Toward an Evidence-Based Approach in Your Own Practice

The following steps are suggested for physicians who want to incorporate an
evidence-based approach into their practice style and clinical decision making:[18]

1. Keep track of clinical questions for follow-up either that day or over the next
   several days.
2. Become aware of what is available through existing print and electronic resources.
3. Subscribe to *Evidence-Based Medicine* (1-800-523-1546) or its CD-ROM, *Best
   Evidence* (1-800-523-1546, extension 2600, or 215-351-2600).
4. Increase your reading of predigested information within your specialty or interest areas.
5. Meet with a librarian at your nearest health sciences library to arrange a tutorial
   in current search tools, such as PubMed.
6. Establish Web sites on your office and/or home computer for useful sources of
   evidence-based abstracts and reports.
7. Seek out consultants who value and rolemodel evidence-based approaches in
   their practices.
8. Reorient your continuing medical education (CME) to evidence-based courses
   as they become more available.

Strengths and Limitations of Evidence-Based Medicine

It seems clear that on occasions like those illustrated in Scenarios 1 and 3, the
strengths of evidence-based medicine are confirmed in answering clinical questions in a timely and useful way in the care of individual patients. As the trends continue toward more extensive use of electronic and print predigested (secondary)
sources of information, we can reasonably expect that EBM will play a stronger
role in everyday clinical decision making. Sackett and his colleagues offer the following rationale for adopting EBM principles in medical education and practice:[19]

1. Increasingly available new evidence can and should lead to major changes in
   patient care.

2. Practicing physicians often fail to obtain available relevant evidence.
3. A practioner's medical knowledge and clinical performance deteriorate with time.
4. Traditional CME is inefficient and generally does not improve clinical performance.
5. Evidence-based medicine can keep the physician up to date.

The gathering momentum of evidence-based medicine is illustrated by several markers of its progress. The U.S. Preventive Services Task Force has established a widely quoted model for the rigorous assessment of the quality and value of evidence—and they base their recommendations on the strength of available evidence.[20] The Cochrane Collaboration now includes more than 1,000 investigators around the world, and they have completed rigorous review of more than 1,000 clinical topics; more than 200 new reviews are added each year and all are updated as necessary. In addition to the Cochrane Database of Systematic Reviews (CDSR), the Cochrane Library also contains the Database of Abstracts of Reviews of Effectiveness (DARE) and the Controlled Clinical Trials Register (CCTR). Two studies in the United Kingdom have shown relevance to conditions seen in everyday practice. One found that 81% of interventions in a suburban training general practice were based on randomized controlled trial (RCT) evidence or convincing nonexperimental evidence,[21] while another study on a general medical ward showed that 82% of treatments were evidence-based (53% with RCT support and 29% with convincing nonexperimental evidence).[22]

The need is obvious for more time-efficient methods for busy clinicians to incorporate updated clinical knowledge into their daily practice. One direct-observation study of physicians showed that an average of two questions were raised for every two or three patient encounters.[23] *The Physicians' Desk Reference,* by no means evidence-based, is thought by many to be the most common reference used by clinicians in their daily schedule. Approximately two-thirds of questions generated during patient encounters are not answered.[23]

Although the evidence-based approach is gaining favor and influence, it has many limitations. A fundamental problem is that many, even most, questions about the diagnosis, natural history, treatment, and outcomes of care for many conditions seen regularly in primary care practice will never be the subjects of the present gold standard of evidence—the RCT. The Cochrane Collaboration has so far confined itself to RCT evidence, so it is not prepared to assess potentially valid evidence based on nonexperimental studies. In a thoughtful paper, Edwards and his colleagues called attention to this problem, noted that many "weaker" study designs are also credible and valid, and proposed the following hierarchy for assessment of type and strength of evidence:[24]

1. Systematic reviews and meta-analysis of randomized trials
2. Well-designed randomized trials
3. Well-designed trials without randomization (e.g., single-group pre-post, cohort, time series, or matched case-controlled studies)
4. Well-designed nonexperimental studies from more than one center
5. Opinions of respected authorities, based on clinical evidence, descriptive studies, or reports of expert committees

There are other limitations with evidence-based medicine in its present state of development. Time constraints and the pressure of everyday practice, of course, require information retrieval techniques to be expeditious and user friendly. Many clinicians are not yet skilled in the methods of critical appraisal of the literature and methods of evidence-based medicine. Many physicians do not yet regularly use the computer for clinical information retrieval. A 1997 study by the American Academy of Family Physicians, for example, found that only 26 percent of U.S. family physicians who have office computers use them for Medline searches.[25] A study of the Medline searches from 1966 to January 1998 revealed that most searches retrieved only one fourth to one half of the relevant articles. Overall use of information retrieval systems was found to be only 0.3 to 9 times per physician per month compared to two unanswered questions for every three patient encounters; even so, it was unclear how these articles were interpreted or applied.[26] Another recent study found that medicine-specific search engines on the World Wide Web performed poorly compared to general search engines, such as MD Consult, Excite, Hot Bot, and Hardin MD.[27] Concerning the most useful kinds of articles—those with POEMs—Ebell and his colleagues recently found that only 2.6 percent of over 8,000 articles of potential interest to primary care physicians in 85 medical journals reported information qualifying as POEMs.[28] Further, and perhaps most important, even the best of evidence-based clinical information still is only a part of what the physician needs in the care of patients—clinical experience and judgment necessarily remain the foundation on which clinical decisions can be individualized to each patient's needs and preferences, often in the context of multiple medical conditions and conflicting priorities.

As hard as it is to generate good evidence, it has been harder to translate this evidence into improving the quality of practice and outcomes, an insight made by Archie Cochrane some time ago that motivated Iain Chalmers and others to try to do so. Although not plentiful, there are a few reports of successful efforts to integrate EBM seamlessly at the point of care.[22,29-30] This involves much more than just access to information, a point that is shown in Table 6.3, which summarizes the five steps necessary to practice evidence-based medicine together with a "plus-minus-zero scorecard" estimating how well we have succeeded in implementing each step in actual practice.[11] Each of these steps need to be considered by proponents of EBM.

The first premise of this assessment is that great progress has been made, and we are perhaps doing best at (+/+) teaching people how to more critically assess the strengths and weaknesses of a variety of different kinds of published or un-

TABLE 6.3 Five steps necessary to practice EBM with a "plus, minus, zero scorecard" for how well we are doing

1. Convert need for information into a clinically relevant, answerable question. (+/−)
2. Efficiently find the best evidence. (+/+/−)
3. Critically appraise the evidence. (+/+)
4. Integrate appraisal with clinical expertise and apply to clinical practice. (+/− /0)
5. Evaluate performance (and outcome). (+/− /0/0)

Source: Adapted from Straus & Sackett[19] and Wolf.[17]

published reports. These reports focus on treatment or prevention effectiveness, the quality of diagnostic tests, prognosis, review articles, clinical practice guidelines, and so on. Training in assessment skills is becoming more prevalent and is typically modeled after the program first developed at McMaster University.[31] Most training uses the *JAMA* critical appraisal series of articles, although the earlier *CMAJ series* and newer *BMJ series* are helpful resources as well.

The second premise is that we are doing almost as well (although not perfectly) at efficiently finding the best evidence $(+/+/-)$. The quality of primary and secondary databases has improved, and improved search strategies have been developed, tested, and even built into some databases like MEDLINE as "EBM filters." Next best $(+/-)$ is our ability to convert the need for information into a clinically relevant, answerable question. This is still something many trainees and seasoned professionals alike struggle with; the difficulty of framing a question such that evidence can be sought to answer it can be deceptive. Finally, it can be argued that we are doing less well $(+/-/0)$ at integrating our appraisal of the evidence with clinical expertise in applying the evidence to clinical practice and even worse $(+/-/0/0)$ at evaluating our performance and documenting the outcomes of applying evidence in our care of patients.[11]

Future Directions in the Information Age

We appear to be entering into what could loosely be called the "brave new world of evidence-based life."[11] The increasing ubiquitousness of evidence-based and "pseudo" evidence-based life, or better put, information-based (overloaded) life, is apparent. The U.S. President's Information Technology Advisory Committee Interim Report (August 1998) estimated that the number of computers connected to the Internet is doubling every year and that the number of people using the Internet worldwide exceeded 100 million people in 1997. This is projected to increase to over 1 billion people by 2005. Bill Gates applauds the "digital nervous system," where information is available on demand, anywhere, at any time, by anyone. Communication will become increasingly seamless and automated between and among all the players or stakeholders in healthcare, as well as in all aspects of life. Wireless and handheld (or pocket-sized) devices are becoming more commonplace, and an increasing variety of toolkits tailored to specific user and audience needs are appearing. There will be better and more megadatabases and multisource "evidence-specific" search engines that really work. Electronic communication between physicians is increasing rapidly and leading to changes in the process of everyday clinical practice. More physician groups and even some solo practitioners are adopting one or another form of electronic medical records, to which clinical practice guidelines and evidence-based protocols can be readily added.

The challenge is to be cognizant of the shortcomings, not just the benefits, of all the new electronic gadgets and tools. As the amount of useful information and high-quality clinical evidence becomes more plentiful and easier to access by everyone, it is important to use it wisely. Patients and the public will increasingly go to their physicians with the latest information they can find on the Internet. Health professionals will need to be able to ascertain the quality of this information and distinguish real evidence from pseudo evidence and justify assessments with valid evidence. It may become important for physicians to be able to access the Internet in real time to quickly review this information firsthand alone or even together with their patients. If they don't do this, patients may be driven away toward more receptive physicians, which may not be in the long-term interest of providing the highest quality of care to patients. High-quality evidence, along with professional experience and expertise, and patient preferences and choices all need to be incorporated into the process of making more informed decisions. New advances and improvements in technology and informatics will contribute to augmenting the speed and value of this process while improving the quality of care in a new relationship with patients.

Glossary of Terms

absolute risk reduction (risk difference)   To estimate the absolute risk reduction (ARR), simply subtract the risk from one group from that of the other rather than take the ratio of the risks for the two groups (the relative risk reduction). The absolute risk reduction is also sometimes referred to as the risk difference. For the example in Scenario 2, we calculate the following:

$$\text{Risk (Mammography)} = 71/58,148 = 0.00122$$
$$\text{Risk (Controls)} = 76/41,104 = 0.00185$$
$$\text{Absolute risk reduction (Risk difference)} = 0.00122 - 0.000185 = -0.06\%$$

Thus the absolute reduction in deaths from breast cancer in our example is 0.06%.

Best Evidence   CD that contains full-text articles from *ACP Journal Club* and the journal *Evidence-Based Medicine,* each of which summarizes recently published articles reporting clinical trials or systematic reviews with a commentary on clinical applicability.

Cochrane Collaboration   "The Cochrane Collaboration is an international network of individuals and institutions committed to preparing, maintaining, and disseminating systematic reviews of the effects of health care. In pursuing its aims, the Cochrane Collaboration is guided by six principles: collaboration, building on people's existing enthusiasm and interests, minimizing duplication of effort, avoidance of bias, keeping up to date, and ensuring access." (hiru.mcmaster *.ca/COCHRANE*)

Cochrane Library   The Cochrane Library contains several databases, including CDSR (Cochrane Database of Systematic Reviews), DARE (the Database of Abstracts of Reviews of Effectiveness of non-Cochrane produced systematic reviews), and CCTR (Controlled Clinical Trials Register).

evidence-based medicine (EBM)   EBM is a "a process of lifelong, self-directed learning in which caring for our own patients creates the need for clinically important information about diagnosis, prognosis, therapy and other clinical and health care issues . . . [that] requires a bottom-up approach that integrates the best external evidence with individual clinical expertise and patient choice."[6]

meta-analysis "Meta-analysis refers to the analysis of analyses . . . the statistical analysis of a large collection of analysis results from individual studies for the purpose of integrating the findings. It connotes a rigorous alternative to the casual, narrative discussions of research studies which typify our attempts to make sense of the rapidly expanding research literature." (Glass, *Educational Researcher,* 1976)

number needed to treat (or screen)   Number of patients needed to be treated (commonly abbreviated NNT) or screened to prevent one adverse outcome (e.g, death) is simply the inverse of the absolute risk reduction (or risk difference).

Absolute risk reduction (ARR) = 0.00122 − 0.00185 = −0.00063 (0.06%)
Number needed to treat (NNT) = 1/(ARR)
$$NNT = 1/0.00063 = 1{,}588$$

Thus 1588 people need to be screened to prevent one breast cancer-specific death. The NNT can be adjusted for the underlying risk group that is most representative of a particular patient's characteristics and risk were the patient to be untreated (or receive standard care).

odds ratio   Here we estimate the odds of an adverse event for each group by dividing the number of adverse events for each group by the number of people not experiencing the adverse event in that group and then taking the ratio of these odds to estimate the odds ratio. The reduction in odds is simply 1 minus the odds ratio. For the example in Scenario 2,

Odds dying (mammography) = 71/58,077 = 0.00122
Odds dying (controls) = 76/41,028 = 0.00185
Odds ratio = 0.00122/0.00185 = 0.659
Odds reduction = 1 = 0.659 = 0.341 = 34%

Thus it is estimated that mammography screening reduced the odds of breast cancer-specific death by 34% over a 7-year period. This breast cancer screening example illustrates the special case in which the risk and odds are identical. This only occurs when the number of events is small and the sample sizes are large for both groups. This is because it matters not whether the number of events (e.g., deaths) in patients randomized to one group or another (e.g., mammography group) is divided by the total number of people in that group (to calculate relative risk) or by the total number of people who did not experience the vent (i.e., were still living), since these numbers are both large and tend to approximate each other.

POEMs   POEMs (Patient-Oriented Evidence that Matters) are synopses of clinically relevant articles, and are contrasted to DOEs (Disease Oriented Evidence). They are published on a Web site under the auspices of the *Journal of Family Practice.*

relative risk reduction   To determine the relative risk, divide (or take the ratio of) the risk of an adverse outcome for people randomized to one group by the risk of an adverse event for people randomized to the other group, and then subtract the result from 1 to estimate the reduction in relative risk. For the example in Scenario 2, the following 2 × 2 table can be constructed.

2 × 2 table for Scenario 2 that summarizes breast cancer-specific survival at seven-year follow-up for women >50 years of age with and without mammography screening (based on Tabar et al., 1985)

Group	Dead	Alive	Total
Mammography	71	58,077	58,148
Controls	76	41,028	41,104
			99,252

$$\text{Risk (mammography)} = 71/58{,}148 = 0.00122$$
$$\text{Risk (controls)} = 76/41{,}104 = 0.00185$$
$$\text{Relative risk (RR)} = 0.00122/0.00185 = 0.659$$
$$\text{RR reduction} = 1 - 0.659 = 0.341 = 34\%$$

Thus mammography screening can be estimated to reduce rate of breast cancer specific death by 34% over a 7-year period.

survival rates differences   For each group, we divide the number of patients *not* experiencing the adverse event by the total number of people in that group and take the difference in these rates between the two groups. For the example in Scenario 2, we find

$$\text{Survival rate (mammography)} = 58{,}077/58{,}148 = 0.9988 = 99.88\%$$
$$\text{Survival rate (controls)} = 41{,}028/41{,}104 = 0.9982 = 99.8\%$$

Thus mammography screening increased the rate of patients surviving from breast cancer from 99.82% to 99.88% over a seven-year period.

systematic review   "Use of this term implies only that a review has been prepared using some kind of systematic approach to minimizing biases and random errors, and that the components of the approach will be documented in a materials and methods section."[32]

TRIP   TRIP (Translating Research into Practice) is a Web site that provides a simple search mechanism for an "amalgamation of 26 databases of hyperlinks from 'Evidence-based' sites around the world." (homepage. http://www.tripdatabase.com/)

References

1. Heidenreich PA, McDonald KM, Hastie T, et al. Meta-analysis of trials comparing beta-blockers, calcium antagonists, and nitrates for stable angina. *JAMA* 1999;281:1927–36.

2. Wennberg J. Dealing with medical practice variations: a proposal for action. *Health Aff Millwood* 1984;3(2):6–32.
3. Kuhn TS. *The Structure of Scientific Revolutions*. Chicago, University of Chicago Press, 1970.
4. Evidence-Based Working Group. Evidence-based medicine: A new approach to teaching the practice of medicine. *JAMA* 1992;268:2420–5.
5. Rosenberg W, Donald A. Evidence-based medicine: an approach to clinical problem-solving. *BMJ* 1995;310:1122–6.
6. Sackett DL, Rosenberg WM, Gray JA, Haynes RB, Richardson WS. Evidence-based medicine: What it is and what it isn't. *BMJ* 1996;312:71–2.
7. Haynes RB, Sackett DL, Gray JA, Cook DJ, Guyatt GH. Transferring evidence from research into practice. 1. The role of clinical care research evidence in clinical decisions. *ACP J Club* 1996;125:A14–16.
8. Slawson DC, Shaughnessy AF, Bennett JH. Becoming a medical information master: Feeling good about not knowing everything. *J Fam Pract* 1994;38:505–13.
9. Shaughnessy AF, Slawson DC, Bennett JH. Becoming an information master: A guidebook to the medical information jungle. *J Fam Pract* 1994;39:489–99.
10. Ebell M. Information at the point of care: Answering clinical questions. *J Am Board Fam Pract* 1999;12:225–35.
11. Wolf FM. Lessons to be learned from evidence-based medicine: Practice and promise of evidence-based medicine and evidence-based education. *Medical Teacher 2000;* 22(3):251–259.
12. TRIP (Translating Research into Practice) homepage. http://www.tripdatabase.com/
13. Tabar L, Fagerberg CJ, Gad A, et al. Reduction in mortality from breast cancer after mass screening with mammography. Randomised trial from the Breast Cancer Screening Working Group of the Swedish National Board of Health and Welfare. *Lancet* 1985;1:829–32.
14. Fahey T, Griffiths S, Peters TJ. Evidence-based purchasing: Understanding results of clinical trials and systematic reviews. *BMJ* 1995;311:1056–60.
15. Wolf FM. Using evidence of effectiveness from randomized trials and meta-analyses to make health care decisions: How information is framed may affect judgments. (Abstract). *Med Decis Making* 1996;16:464.
16. Wolf FM. Interpreting results of RCTs and meta-analyses: implications for providers, consumers, and policy makers. (Abstract) Proceedings of the 5th International Cochrane Colloquium, Amsterdam, The Netherlands, October 1997, p. 240.
17. Wolf FM. Summarizing evidence for clinical use. In: Geyman JP, Deyo RA, Ramsey SD, eds. *Evidence-based Clinical Practice: Concepts and Approaches*. Woburn, MA: Butterworth-Heinemann, 2000, pp. 133–43.
18. Geyman JP. Evidence-based medicine in primary care: An overview. *J Am Board Fam Pract* 1998;11:46–56.
19. Sackett DL. *Evidence-based medicine: How to practice and teach EBM*. 2nd ed. New York: Churchill Livingstone, 1997, pp. 2–16.

20. US Preventive Services Task Force Staff. *The guide to clinical preventive services: Report of the United States Preventive Services Task Force.* 2nd ed. Philadelphia: Williams & Wilkins, 1996, pp. 861–2.
21. Gill P, Dowell AC, Neal RD, Smith N, Heywood P, Wilson AE. Evidence-based general practice: A retrospective study of interventions in one training practice. *BMJ* 1996;312:819–21.
22. Ellis J, Mulligan I, Rowe J, Sackett DL. Inpatient general medicine is evidence based. *Lancet* 1995;346:407–10.
23. Covell DG, Uman GC, Manning PR. Information needs in office practice: Are they being met? *Ann Intern Med* 1985:103:596–99.
24. Edwards AK, Russell IT, Stott NC. Signal versus noise in the evidence base for medicine: An alternative to hierarchies of evidence? *Fam Pract* 1998;15(4): 319–22.
25. Is anyone using computerized records? *Fam Pract Management* 1977;4(4):96.
26. Hersh WR, Hickam DH. How well do physicians use electronic information retrieval systems? A framework for investigation and systematic review. *JAMA* 1998;280:1347–52.
27. Graber MA, Bergus GR, York C. Using the World Wide Web to answer clinical questions: How efficient are different methods of information retrieval? *J Fam Pract* 1999;48:520–4.
28. Ebell MH, Barry HC, Slawson DC, Shaughnessy AF. Finding POEMs in the medical literature. *J Fam Pract* 1999;48:350–5.
29. Cates C. An evidence-based approach to reducing antibiotic use in children with acute otitis media: Controlled before and after study. *BMJ* 1999;318: 715–6.
30. Shaughnessy AF, Slawson DC. Are we providing doctors with the training and tools for lifelong learning? *BMJ* 1999;319:1280.
31. Oxman AD, Sackett DL, Guyatt G. Users' guides to the medical literature: I. How to get started. *JAMA* 1993;270:2093–5.
32. Glass, G.V. Primary, secondary and meta-analysis of research. Educational Research 1976;5:3–8.
33. Chambers I, Altman DG. Systematic Reviews. London, BMJ Publishing Group, 1995.

7
Clinical Decision Support

PETER TARCZY-HORNOCH, M.D. AND THOMAS H. PAYNE, M.D.

Scenario 1

A 2-year-old girl is brought to a small rural emergency room at ten o'clock at night by her babysitter who found her in the bathroom with an open unlabeled container of her grandfather's heart pills. The general pediatrician on call for the ER needs to identify the pills, determine what diagnostic workup is necessary, and initiate appropriate treatment. If unswallowed pills are unavailable the pediatrician might try to contact the grandfather's physician to determine what medications he is taking. In the future, the pediatrician might access the grandfather's electronic medical record through emergency override.

Today, a common response for a clinician faced with possible poisoning is to contact a poison control center to receive information over the phone and/or via fax regarding management of possible overdose of each medication. Electronic resources are already available and becoming more prevalent that will greatly augment this phone call to the poison control center. There are electronic tools to aid in identification of unknown pills via color, size, shape, manufacturer, and imprints. These resources save tremendous time compared to the manual or phone alternative. The electronic documents used by poison control centers are now available directly to practitioners. Full text versions of textbooks, journals, and other diagnostic tools are becoming available on line, including adult and pediatric emergency room textbooks that contain sections on managing possible poisoning with unknown agents as well as specific agents. Third-party companies (information aggregators, information mediators) are pulling together these disparate resources so that from a single Web page the pediatrician will be able to access a very rich library and toolkit of resources at ten o'clock at night (in this case to identify the pills, identify general poisoning management and workup, and identify medication-specific poisoning management and workup). A caveat is that such resources will not replace the pediatrician's need to talk late at night with a person more experienced with poisoning that she is. Thus, an alternate scenario for this hypothetical situation is the expansion of the electronic library available to the poison control center.

Scenario 2

A physician making weekend hospital rounds for her group practice is about to see an elderly male admitted the previous day by her colleague for fever following chemotherapy. She uses a mobile laptop that rolls on a cart with a wireless connection to the patient's electronic record to read the admission note and a recently completed nursing note and to review the patient's chest film image while at the patient's bedside. She is paged with a message from the hospital clinical computing system reporting that that the hematocrit on a patient she saw earlier has returned. The message indicates that while the result is still in the normal range, it has dropped 8 points since the previous night, suggesting recurrent hemorrhage and the need for reevaluation and transfusion. Using her workstation, she orders blood products, alerts the nurse caring for the patient that a transfusion is planned, and writes a brief addendum to her progress note to reflect this important new development. Responding to the page, writing the note and orders, and calling the nurse required 3 minutes. Returning to the review of her mobile workstation screen, she sees an alert that sensitivities on a blood culture from the patient she is about to see have just returned. They indicate that the organism is not sensitive to the empirical antibiotics with which the patient is currently being treated. She confirms that the patient has had an allergic reaction after receiving a cephalosporin and writes an order for trimethoprim/sulfamethoxazole, which is on the hospital formulary and available. Before signing the order, a prompt appears apprising her that the patient received a single dose of methotrexate last evening, and this may interact with trimethoprim/sulfamethoxazole. She cancels the order, orders a different drug proposed by the order entry application, and signs it. She spends the next 15 minutes talking with and examining her patient and then continues rounds, which she completes before lunch. That afternoon she follows the progress of her patients and reviews new laboratory results by consulting the electronic record from her home workstation.

Background

Scenarios 1 and 2 illustrate a spectrum of clinician information needs at the point of care. The information is needed to inform clinical decisions in a very specific context, namely a particular patient with a particular set of issues at a particular point in time. Many studies (an overview of which is provided in the readings) have examined clinician information needs at the point of care and have found that they can broadly be divided into patient-specific information (e.g., the medical record) and medical knowledge. Some needs are clearly patient specific (what drugs is a patient currently taking?), others are more clearly related to medical knowledge (what are the side effects of this new drug I am considering prescribing?), and others sit at the intersection (what might the adverse interactions be between this new drug I am about to prescribe and the drugs my patient is already taking?). Currently in the paper world, these information needs are frequently unmet (the conservative estimate is at least one unmet information need per patient-provider encounter; see the article by Smith in Recommended Readings).

The fact that information is in paper form contributes to the inaccessibility of the information—a paper document (medical record, textbook, guideline) is by definition in a single location and can't be shared simultaneously, unlike an electronic document, which can be accessed simultaneously from multiple locations. Thus, in the absence of electronic resources, a clinician on call at home has no access to the patient's record (which is at the clinic) and typically has access to a very limited subset of medical knowledge resources (most are at the office). In the primary care practitioner's patient exam room, the patient record is available (barring missing data such as lab results not yet filed, details regarding a recent hospitalization, and so on), but access to knowledge resources is limited (they are down the hall or in the library). Electronic clinical decision support tools integrated with electronic record systems have the potential to streamline access to information at the point of care (the concept of "just-in-time" information), which by extension has the potential to improve patient care (shown in limited respects by some studies).

Some important additional challenges posed by paper-based medical record systems are discussed in Chapter 10 (Workflow Automation), Chapter 4 (Importing Laboratory Data), and Chapter 2 (Electronic Medical Record). Some challenges especially germane to clinical decision making at the point of care include timeliness and currency of paper-based resources and incorporating institution-specific information with reference materials, both of which are difficult using paper media.

Challenges posed by paper-based sources of medical knowledge are addressed in Chapter 6 (Evidence-Based Medicine), Chapter 8 (Knowledge Resources), and Chapter 9 (Patient Education Resources and Instruction). Some issues particularly germane to clinical decision making at the point of care are highlighted here. Peer-reviewed journals, though authoritative and timely, are not designed to provide an up-to-date synopsis of clinical issues for use at the point of care. Textbooks, though excellent synopses of what is known at the time of publication, degrade in terms of information currency the farther away they are from the publication date. Additionally, they are typically subject to neither peer review nor rigorous standards of evidence. Review articles in peer-reviewed journals to some extent combine currency, synopsis, and peer review but in print format are not organized for easy context-specific retrieval (when seeing a patient with refractory hypertension, you want the most recent peer-reviewed review articles on hypertension from a list of preferred journals, not an article on some other topic from this month's journal). To address the need for high-quality, synthesized, evidence-based material, a number of groups have started to develop resources summarizing the current state of the evidence (such as the Cochrane Collaboration—see the article by Bero and Rennie in Recommended Readings and the *British Medical Journal*). However, electronic access at the point of care to these resources does not solve the entire problem, because these resources were not designed and structured to be used quickly and efficiently to answer specific questions at the point of care. The one class of paper resources designed to provide just-in-time point-of-care information is the pocket manuals and guides frequently used by junior house staff. These resources do meet the need for information, though frequently they do not provide sufficient detail for more esoteric or complex questions such as those encountered in practice by experienced clinicians.

Decision Support and the Clinician

The most suitable time to help clinicians make a decision is the moment the decision must be made. This requires that decision support functions be present with the clinician as the work is being performed. We care for patients during clinic visits, hospital rounds, in the emergency room, and when answering telephone calls (or increasingly, reading and answering e-mail). Since computer-based decision support requires access to some form of computer, then the computer or other electronic device must be easily accessible to the clinician when delivering care.

Convenient access to a computing device can be accomplished by positioning desk-based workstations in locations accessible during rounds or clinic encounters or by arranging for the device to be carried or rolled along with the clinician. Wireless network technologies now make this practical and safe. High-frequency, low-power transceivers can be safely used next to patient monitoring equipment.

There is rapid change in the kinds of devices used in patient care. Traditionally, desk-based or wall-mounted workstations were the norm, often with large monitors to allow viewing large grids containing patient results and images. Though such workstations remain common, they are being supplemented with mobile and hand-held devices. The mix of size and mobility of devices will change with technological advances, but one principle will remain: to take full advantage of the ability for computing systems to influence decisions, they need to be used at the time decisions are made.

Another critical element of workflow is the speed with which work is performed. Time for clinic visits, hospital rounds, and other activities is short and becoming shorter. Decisions must be made quickly, and because of this physicians may make decisions in the absence of full information. The need for speed may influence how frequently clinicians turn to decision support resources and how much time they spend entering patient information into the decision support resource when it is used.

Decision Support Techniques

Computing systems can help clinicians make decisions in a variety of ways. Gathering and displaying laboratory results to make trends obvious, allowing rapid review of consultant notes and discharge summaries, and giving access to all these information sources wherever needed—in the office, at home, at the bedside—is an extremely powerful form of decision support.

As the volume of information needed to practice healthcare increases, automated review of the information to generate prompts and reminders is not only possible but critical so that needed care is not overlooked: Printed or screen displays generated by simple rules have long been recognized as an effective means of improving care quality.

In some arenas, detailed patient information is gathered in a form that allows computing systems to conduct more rigorous analysis and to generate hypotheses or treatment recommendations. Some of these systems exhibit characteristics we label as intelligence; the term artificial intelligence is applied to this area of automated decision support. These systems include differential diagnoses drawn from analysis of a large set of individual patient data and a large knowledge base of diseases and syndromes. Sometimes very detailed treatment plans are generated by artificial intelligence systems.

The convergence of large medical knowledge bases and detailed patient databases containing information in a form that can be "understood" by computing systems makes possible all these forms of decision support. There are many approaches to generating the advice or recommendations that the clinician ultimately views.

One can think of decision support systems along a spectrum ranging from tools to facilitate patient care (analogous to a word processor facilitating document creation) to sophisticated systems that attempt to replicate the behavior of expert clinicians (analogous to a chess-playing computer). The term "decision support system" in the medical informatics literature typically refers to the more sophisticated of these systems.

Brief descriptions of some of the underlying approaches used by different systems follow. Selected references are provided for more information. For the practicing clinician the important point to keep in mind is that a variety of theoretical foundations underlie existing commercial decision support systems. Each approach has its strengths and weaknesses. The performance of a given system, however, depends not only on the underlying model but also on the quality of the information used to develop the model—the computer jargon term GIGO ("garbage in, garbage out") summarizes this aspect nicely.

Mathematical Modeling

In a limited number of domains mathematical models have been developed for clinical decision support purposes. A familiar class of mathematical models widely used in clinical practice are pharmacokinetic models. These form the basis for nomograms and equations used to adjust drug dosages based on measured drug levels and/or function of end organs (e.g., renal clearance). Mathematical models are not widely used since often there are insufficient data to develop a rigorous model. Furthermore, mathematical models are often complex and cannot be readily used to explain to the clinician user how a recommendation made by the decision support system was derived.

Rule Based Systems

A number of terms are used to describe systems essentially driven by a series of rules, including expert systems, AI systems, and rule based systems. These systems attempt to capture in a variety of ways the decision-making process of experts in a field (either diagnostic or therapeutic). Simple rule based systems are frequently used to prevent errors (e.g., IF <drug__prescribed>ELEMENT__OF <drugs__patient__allergic__to>THEN <alert__clinician>). A starting point for a more sophisticated rule based system can be an algorithm, a flowchart, or a guideline that is then converted to a more formal notation that can be used by a computerized system to replicate elements of more sophisticated decision making by an expert. A classic example of such a system is the MYCIN expert system used to empirically choose antibiotic therapy for suspected infection. A major strength of rule based decision support systems is their ability to explain to the clinician user the logical chain that led to a conclusion or recommendation by the system. A limitation of classic rule based systems is the absence of a good way to represent uncertainty and probability (e.g., most of the time if A then B but sometimes C). Simple rule based systems for alerts, reminders, error checking, and similar applications are relatively widely used. More sophisticated rule based systems are less often used—in part because of the challenges in maintaining a large, complex set of rules.

Decision Analysis

Decision analysis is a formal mathematical and statistical approach designed to arrive at an optimal decision given a set of constraints and in the face of uncertainty. Decision analyses are used relatively frequently in the medical literature to arrive at guidelines and recommendations for preventive care measures. Decision analysis takes into account the "cost" of the preventive measure, the incidence of the condition to be prevented, the probability of the condition to be prevented occurring with and without the preventive measure, and the "cost" of the condition occurring. A number of decision support systems use more complex decision analysis models to guide clinicians and/or patients through complex decision pathways—particularly where the expected value of a treatment may vary from patient to patient. These more complex models involve multiple levels of decisions, each with multiple outcomes represented in a graph or tree structure.

Bayesian Statistics

Bayesian statistics are another formal statistical approach to representing and handling uncertainty in clinical decision making. A simple use of the Bayes theorem is to update the probability of a diagnosis in response to a test result after taking into account the prior probability of the diagnosis (often starting with the prevalence of the disease in the population) and characteristics of the test itself (sensitivity and specificity). A number of decision support systems use more complex Bayesian systems that rely on what is known as a belief network. A belief network permits representing multiple interlinked observations and their impact on one another and the probability of one or more outcomes of interest.

Active Decision Support

We define "active" decision support as support brought to the attention of the clinician without being requested. Windows, dialog boxes, or screens are presented automatically and at the appropriate time—when writing orders or documenting care, for example. Usually the information presented is brief, immediately relevant to the task at hand and offers more detailed information if desired. Examples of this form of decision support are reminders and prompts, order checks invoked during the order entry process, and event-based notification.

Reminders are among the longest-standing forms of clinical computing decision support and still are among the most effective. They typically appear to remind the clinician of the need for an intervention, such as an immunization, at the time of a clinic visit or appointment. To speed performance they may be generated in advance and displayed at the time of the visit. They may be printed on paper or appear on the screen or on a pager. Usually the reminder includes text that justifies its appearance for that patient at that time, such as a listing of prior immunizations or the diagnoses leading to the recommendation for immunization.

Order checks are screens that appear during the ordering process. A prompt may appear in a small screen when a medication to which the patient is allergic is ordered or to flag an important interaction between medication the patient is taking and the agent being ordered. Usually order checks rely on rapid comparison of patient-specific data, such as known allergies or current medications, with a large table of drug-drug, drug-allergy, drug-laboratory, or drug-diagnosis information. These tables may be produced and maintained by a vendor or by pharmacists within the organization. Order checks are among the most important forms of decision support available. They are common features of computing systems used by pharmacists.

One of the challenges to those who implement clinical computing systems is to assure that prompts that convey the most important information are used but that those that convey less important information are not. If too many prompts appear for less than critical reasons, clinicians may either begin to ignore the prompts or lobby for them to be removed from the system. An example of prompts that are less valuable are alerts at the time of medication renewal that the patient is allergic to a medication the patient has been taking without problem for the past two weeks.

An event-based alert, broadly defined, is generated when a prespecified "rule" or short program is run at the time that an event occurs. Triggering events may be registration or admission of a patient, availability of a new laboratory result, entry of a specific order type, or the passage of a specified amount of time since a prior event. Applications that create event-based alerts are often called "event monitors," because they monitor clinical computing systems in use in the healthcare organization to determine when alerts should be run. Event-based alerts may be triggered by some external process, or by a clinician's action.

Developing the logic or set of rules that are at the heart of active decision support systems is a difficult and time-consuming task. First, there needs to be agreement on the general approach the logic will take. This may require literature review, meetings with local or national experts, or a combination of approaches for developing clinical guidelines. In some cases—for example, that it is important to note that a hematocrit has dropped 8 points—there may be no disagreement with the underlying logic.

Next, the logic or rule needs to be translated into a form that can run on the organizational clinical computing systems. This requires identifying data on which the logic will operate and refining the algorithm so that it performs as desired. When this is accomplished, the logic needs to be extensively tested. Finally, when the logic is put into production, it must be monitored to see that it performs in the real world as it did in the testing environment; often unexpected circumstances require that the logic be modified.

This process must be followed for every active decision support module, and it often takes many years to develop a useful library. To reduce the time to achieve a useful set of decision support rules, sharing of usable sets of logic—sometimes referred to as medical logic modules—has been proposed and tried. One standard for sharing is to express the logic in a standard protocol, such as the Arden syntax. There are small collections of medical logic modules available on the World Wide Web. The degree of sharing is not what was expected when the standard was developed, however. One of the reasons is that computing systems that can take advantage of this logic are not common in healthcare organizations. As clinical computing systems with decision support features are more broadly adopted, medical logic module sharing may become more common.

Examples of Decision Support Systems

Web-Based Clinical Decision Support—GeneClinics

The Web is becoming an important clinical decision support tool for both patients and providers. One of the top uses of the Web (by people who are not healthcare providers) is to find health-related information. Surveys have shown that as many as 80% of the general public have used the Web in a 12-month period to search for health-related information. Provider use of the Web is lagging: an estimated forty percent of providers use the Web at least occasionally to search for medical information. Concern is growing, however, about the quality of the available information that consumers are accessing, and a number of organizations have created guidelines for assessing the quality of medical information on the Web (for example the HON Code Principles—www.hon.ch/HONcode/Conduct.html—of authority, complementarity, confidentiality, attribution, justifiability, transparency of authorship, transparency of sponsorship). The growing adoption of the Web as a source of health-related information is being spurred by the growing ubiquity of access to the Web, the low cost of distribution of information, and the theoretical ability of the Web to maintain currency in a way that the print medium can't.

Decision support tools available on the Web cover the spectrum from electronic versions of material originally developed for print distribution to sophisticated decision support tools specifically developed for distribution via the Web. The principle of "Caveat lector" articulated by the editors of *JAMA* holds true. Users need to assess for themselves the utility, reliability, authoritativeness, currency, and relevance of these tools just as they would assess these factors for a new journal, textbook, or article. The sophisticated decision support tools that interact with the user and make treatment and/or diagnostic suggestions are more difficult to assess, though work has been done in this area. A number of commercial and public-domain Web sites integrate access to a broad range of on-line journals, handbooks, textbooks, and tools. A sample of these types of tools can be seen in the University of Washington Care Provider Toolkit at http://healthlinks.washington .edu/toolkits/care__provider.html (note that access to many of these resources is password restricted). Most of the available decision support tools on the Web were originally developed for use in other environments and then secondarily distributed via the Web. There is a small but growing number of resources that were developed explicitly with point-of-care access via the Web in mind.

The GeneClinics (www.geneclinics.org) expert-written peer-reviewed database of information on the application of genetic testing is an example of a point-of-care Web-based resource that is not a repackaging of an existing print resource (Figure 7.1). The revolution in genetic testing that has resulted from the Human Genome Project to date has created a significant challenge for healthcare providers that extends well beyond clinical geneticists. As the genetic bases for common conditions (such as breast cancer) are identified, primary care providers and other specialists need to have an understanding of the applicability and limitations of genetic testing for specific conditions. The GeneClinics resource seeks to meet this information need via a sophisticated electronic publishing model that blends the authority of the peer-review process with the synthesis inherent in a review article or book chapter while maintaining the currency of a journal. Since one of the intended uses of the GeneClinics database entries is at the point of care, they are structured to quickly provide both a summary of key information as well as ready access to more specific information. The Web is an integral part of this process from solicitation of expert authors to internal and external peer review to final publication via the Web. The Web permits continual updating of the resource as needed and cross-linking entries in the GeneClinics database to other Web-based resources such as support groups, consensus statements, genomic databases, and the primary literature.

CPRS

The Veterans Affairs Computerized Patient Record System (CPRS) is an electronic health record used to review results, documents, and images and to enter

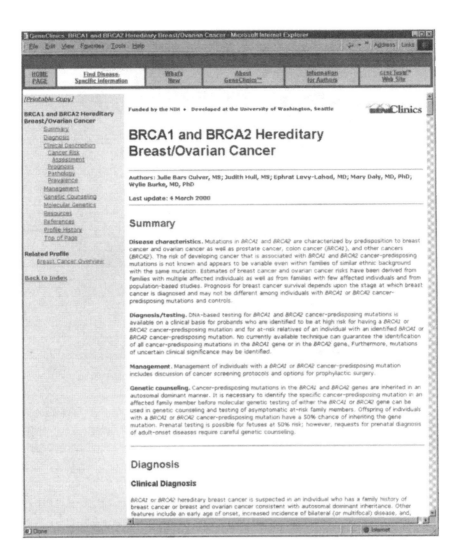

FIGURE 7.1. GeneClinics (www.geneclinics.org) is an example of a point-of-care Web-based resource that is not a repackaging of an existing print resource.

documents and orders. It includes a wide variety of decision support features that are used throughout the process of viewing a patient record.

After the user successfully enters a username and password, a screen appears to allow the patient of interest to be selected. To change patients, this screen must be used. In addition to allowing patient selection, the patient selection screen also displays View Alerts, one-line listings of important information for the attention of the viewing clinician. Examples of View alerts are abnormal laboratory results, orders and notes requiring signature and cosignature, notification of hospital admission or transfer, and other information that pertains to all patients with whom the user has some treating relationship. When a View Alert is selected, CPRS may open to the section of the CPRS record where action (e.g., order signature) should be taken.

When the patient of interest is selected, CPRS usually opens to the Cover Sheet, which displays relevant clinical reminders for that patient. By selecting the reminder, the justification for the reminder is shown, sometimes including a Web site hyperlink. Within the reminder are buttons can that can be used to satisfy the reminder (for example, to order a hemoglobin A1c for a diabetic patient) and document the intervention in two ways: a code is stored for the patient to keep the reminder from showing again until necessary, and a note is started with text inserted documenting what was ordered and for what reason. This feature of the reminders is extremely important: completing all actions needed to satisfy the reminder from within the reminder screen is very fast.

To review laboratory results, the Lab tab is selected. This allows viewing patient results using a traditional display of results in chronological order, but it also allows individual users to prepare worksheets of results pertinent to review of collections of results. For example, to review the effect of lipid-lowering medications, a worksheet might contain all lipid results and liver function tests in a spreadsheet-like format. This saves the time required to dozens of results to search for the LDL cholesterol, for example. The worksheet can be used to display a graph of particular results to quickly ascertain trends that might not be apparent from viewing a listing of results. Graphs are extremely powerful tools for understanding the natural history of disease or long-term treatment progress.

To write orders, the user selects the Orders tab. Orders are usually generated by selecting an order from a screen on which orders for particular clinical scenarios are conveniently grouped. For example, to write orders to begin treatment with patient-controlled analgesia (PCA), there is a screen containing a set of linked orders, called an order set, that can be used to quickly generate all the orders needed. The order set not only orders morphine as the analgesic, it also includes orders for monitoring the patient, medications to treat side effects such as constipation, and it orders a supply of naloxone, a drug used in emergencies to treat narcotic overdose. With one mouse click the clinician can prepare orders for everything needed to begin PCA, including orders that are sometimes omitted. When ordering empirical antibiotics for community-acquired pneumonia, orders can be selected from a screen that both describes treatment options and allows the clinician to order the agent selected (Figure 7.2). This reduces the time required to consult reference materials when writing admission orders for a seriously ill patient.

When orders are submitted for electronic signature, a series of order checks are automatically run to assure there are no duplicate treatments and that the patient has not previously had an allergy or adverse reaction to the agents ordered. These order checks appear in real time and are completed before the order is released to the filling service (for example, a pharmacy). The clinician can override any alert, though in the case of severe drug interaction or allergy, the clinician may be required to enter a justification for the override.

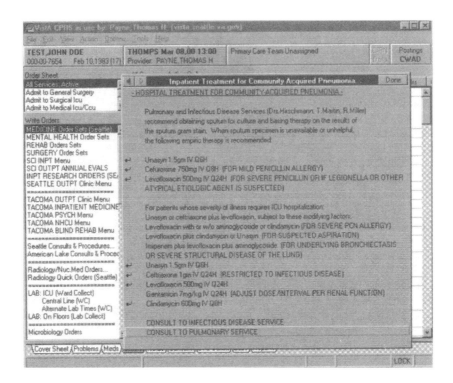

FIGURE 7.2. Ordering screen from CPRS. Treatment recommendations and orders are combined in the CPRS automated record. Clicking on the line describing an antimicrobial agent prepares the order for submission and executes drug-allergy, drug-drug, and other order checks before the order is released to the filling service.

Selection of Empirical Antimicrobials

We will use a common medical decision to provide examples of many of the principles discussed in this chapter. Most clinicians would agree that choosing an antibiotic for a patient with suspected infection before culture results are known—empirical therapy—requires consideration of many factors (Table 7.1). Some factors in the decision can be derived from the literature, some are specific to the patient, and some depend on institutional decisions and experience.

What tools do we have available to aid us in choosing empirical antibiotics? Experienced clinicians rely on their experience and judgment for decisions they encounter frequently, but when the decision is more difficult, most practitioners have access to reference material in textbooks or though the World Wide Web. These sources describe general approaches to treatment of similar patients, but they are sometimes inconvenient to use. Pocket guides are extremely popular because they can be carried and provide current summaries of recommendations for many clinical conditions. However, pocket guides cannot easily account for formulary differences and resistance patterns among institutions.

TABLE 7.1 Sources and types of information needed when deciding on empirical antimicrobial therapy.

Information considered during decision	Source	Pocket reference book	Personal digital assistant	Integrated clinical computing/order entry system
Likely pathogens	Literature	x	x	x
Antimicrobial sensitivies of likely pathogens		x	x	x
Results of clinical trials		x	x	x
Local resistance patterns	Institution			x
Antimicrobial costs			?	x
Local formulary			?	x
Diagnosis	Patient			x
Allergies and sensitivities				x
Renal function				x
Hepatic function				x
Current and past antimicrobial agents				x
Culture results				x
Other considerations				?

Recently, hand-held personal digital assistants (PDAs) can be used to access programs to assist in selection of empirical antibiotics and for many other purposes. Though they may provide less detail than pocket guides and textbooks, PDAs are extremely convenient, contain information of many types, and often are already in the pockets of physicians because they contain schedules and phone numbers. There are two additional advantages of PDA programs: they can be updated daily with recent recommendations, and they have the potential to include an indication of which antimicrobials are on the institutional formulary.

Textbooks, pocket guides, and PDAs are available to all practitioners in the United States for less than several hundred dollars and in some cases for less than $20. However, these sources do not include information important for individual patient care decisions, as listed in Table 7.1. The practitioner must look up or ask the patient to determine allergies, relevant laboratory and microbiology data, and concurrent medications. Gathering all this information may take as long as 25 minutes if it is done manually, and for this reason, not all the information may be gathered. Since much of the information in Table 7.1 exists in machine-processable form in some medical centers, it could be used in conjunction with an expert system to recommend empirical therapy at specific doses for specific patients. Would such a system be helpful if it were available? This question was answered at LDS Hospital by developing such a system and comparing outcomes of patients treated before and after the system was available for ordering antimicrobials (see the article by Evans in Recommended Readings). The results showed that clinical outcomes such as the number of days on antimicrobial therapy, number of adverse drug reactions, and administrative outcomes such as treatment cost were improved. Such comprehensive and integrated decision support systems are not broadly available, but it is clear why there is great interested in them: they help us do a better job caring for our patients.

Decision support systems are available to all practitioners in some form. Our challenge is to adopt those that are practical for us to use today, to recognize the value of more advanced systems, and to strive to use even better decision support systems as they become available to us.

Recommended readings

Berner ES, Webster GD, Shugerman AA, Jackson JR, Algina J, Baker Al, Ball EV, Cobbs CG, Dennis VW, Frenkel EP, et al. Performance of four computer-based diagnostic systems. *N Engl J Med* 1994;330:1792–1796.

Bero L, Rennie D. The Cochrane Collaboration. Preparing, maintaining, and disseminating systematic reviews of the effects of health care. *JAMA* 1995;274:1935–1938.

Evans RS, Pestotnik SL, Classen DC, Clemmer TP, Weaver LK, Orme JF, Lloyd JF, Burke JP. A computer-assisted management program for antibiotics and other antiinfective agents. *N Engl J Med* 1998;338:232–238.

Fuller, S, Ketchell, DS, Tarczy-Hornoch, P, Masuda, D. Integrating knowledge resources at the point of care: opportunities for librarians. *Bull Med Libr Assoc* 1999;87:393–403.

Owens DG, Sox HC. Medical decision-making: Probabilistic medical reasoning. In: Shortliffe EH, Perreault LE, eds. *Medical Informatics: Computer Applications in Health Care and Biomedicine,* 2nd ed. New York: Springer-Verlag, 2001;76–131.

Payne TH, Torell J, Hoey P. *Implementation of the Computerized Patient Record System and Other Clinical Computing Applications at the VA Puget Sound Health Care System.* Proceedings of the Sixth Annual Nicholas E. Davies CPR Recognition Symposium. Bethesda: CPRI-HOST, 2000.

Silberg WM, Lundberg GD, Musacchio RA. Assessing, controlling, and assuring the quality of medical information on the Internet: Caveat lector et viewor— Let the reader and viewer beware. *JAMA* 1997 Apr 16;277(15):1244–1245.

Smith R. What clinical information do doctors need? *BMJ* 1996;313:1062–1068.

Tarczy-Hornoch P, Shannon P, Baskin P, Espeseth M, Pagon RA. GeneClinics: a hybrid text/data electronic publishing model using XML applied to clinical genetic testing. *J Am Med Inform Assoc* 2000;7:267–276.

8
Knowledge Resources: Finding Answers to Primary Care Questions

Debra S. Ketchell, M.L., H.S.L., Leilani St. Anna, M.L.I.S.,
Sherry Dodson, M.L.S., Sarah Safranek, M.L.I.S.,
Terry Ann Jankowski, M.L.S.

Scenario

9:00 A.M. Your clinic day starts with a teenage girl whose blood sugars are elevated and insulin requirements are increased. She reports that her weight is down. You probe and discover that she has been taking Ma-huang for weight control. You believe that the weight loss may not be worth the risk and recommend that she stop taking Ma-huang until a follow-up visit in two weeks. Before her next visit you will review the evidence on the safety of this herbal supplement for adolescent diabetics.

9:20 A.M. Your next patient is a 42-year-old woman who has nearly finished her radiation for stage 2 breast cancer with adjuvant chemotherapy. She tells you that her family is planning a vacation in Belize to celebrate and asks if she should get a hepatitis A vaccination and take any precautions for diarrhea. To answer her concerns you need to determine any contraindications for hepatitis A and considerations about travelers' diarrhea specific to immunosuppressed patients.

9:40 A.M. A 74-year-old man, who is 4 weeks out from a right hip replacement, presents with excruciating lower back pain of 36 hours duration. He describes the pain as burning, searing, and unremitting. You suspect infection but note that he has no fever and his rehabilitation has been progressing normally. He denies dysuria, falls, or trauma to his hip or back. On physical exam, you note erythematous papules that follow the fifth lumbar sensory nerve distribution and you realize that you need to refresh your memory on the skin findings for herpes zoster while you send the patient for lab tests and hip X rays.

10:00 A.M. Next you see a 58-year-old man with left-sided Bell's palsy of 36 hours duration. You know that some physicians prescribe steroids and possibly antiviral medications, but you wonder whether there is evidence that this is any better than watchful waiting.

10:20 A.M. Your next patient is a 72-year-old woman with osteoarthritis of the knees. She is accompanied by her daughter, a lab tech from the hospital, who wants you to give her mother a prescription for one of the new COX-2 inhibitors. She has heard that they cause less GI bleeding. Her mother is concerned that the new drugs will mean more out-of-pocket costs each month. You want to do some research comparing "coxibs" with established NSAIDS with regard to GI bleeding and efficacy in pain control.

10:40 A.M. Next you see a 57-year-old woman for a routine well-woman exam. She is currently on hormone replacement therapy (HRT) and expresses concern about the risk of breast cancer. She has searched the Web and PubMed MEDLINE™ looking for information about the pros and cons of HRT. There is no family history of breast cancer and previous exams and mammograms were normal. You agree that the medical literature is not definitive and recommend that she not discontinue therapy until you can e-mail her a review of the best evidence based on her specific profile.

Your clinic day is shaping up into one of uncommon presentations and patients asking for assistance in interpreting recommendations for long-term health. It reinforces a nagging issue of how to quickly research questions that arise in your practice. Like many primary care providers, you see an average of 6 to 10 patients per clinic half day. Studies indicate that 1 to 6 questions occur from these patient visits. Ely[1] estimated that at least one substantive question arises for every nine patients in primary care if routine drug lookups are excluded. Studies by Gorman[2,3] found that questions pursued in primary care are patient specific and chosen on the belief there is an answer. While primary care providers often feel overwhelmed by the volume of studies published in the medical literature, Lock[4] estimated that only 15% of this body of knowledge is useful in clinical care. Searching for and analyzing high-quality systematic reviews for clinical decision making is time consuming, and thus the busy primary provider usually turns to a textbook on the shelf or a nearby colleague or lets the question go unanswered.

Patients are also inundated by medical information, particularly when prescription drugs and the latest clinical studies are marketed through the mass media. Many patients and their family members browse the Web in search of answers[5] and find a mixed bag of spurious information, commercial advertisements, medical research articles, clinical trials provided by the government, and professional Web sites. A growing number of medical societies and specialty associations offer "consumer friendly" translations of original studies in their publications (e.g., Summary for Patients in the *Annals of Internal Medicine*[6]). The National Library of Medicine produces MEDLINEplus™, a filtered index to health information, and a clinical trials database.[7] Patients expect their care providers to help interpret this conflicting mass of information. Before effectively counseling their patients, primary care providers must be able to find relevant information, filter out the best from the less credible, and judge whether to believe the information that remains in a world where recommendations for clinical practice are constantly changing.[8,9]

Until recently the state of digested knowledge for primary care was characterized by a lack of evidence. New sources (e.g., UpToDate, Clinical Evidence, Cochrane Library of Systematic Reviews, and Bandolier) synthesize the primary literature to put the best available evidence into clinical practice. The ubiquitous availability of the Internet and mobile or handheld digital devices and the simplicity of Web search engines provide effective methods for placing this evidence at the point of care.

This chapter focuses on the types of questions that arise during patient care in the primary care setting and the identification of the best available sources to inform decision making. We illustrate the use of digital information sources, particularly Web and handheld options that offer enhanced, unique, integrated, or more current information than the traditional textbook. We conclude with trends for the future and research projects in progress.

Time, Relevance, and Access

Gorman's[2,3] research on information seeking in primary care concluded that physicians pursue a question when the problem is urgent or if they perceive that there is an answer. Many information needs go unanswered due to time constraints. If questions are recognized and pursued, physicians usually turn first to colleagues and second to pharmacopoeia or textbooks. Unfortunately, information in the provider's head and in the textbook on the shelf may be out of date or incorrect. New information may not have penetrated common practice or information may not be available to deal with uncommon problems. These deficiencies are exacerbated due to the rate of change in medical knowledge. This contextual framework for patient care information seeking is illustrated in Figure 8.1.

Many questions remain unrecognized, not pursued, and unanswered that could be answered through digital information sources, but it requires time and demands skills that many providers do not possess.[10,11] Alper[12] found that over 60% of common questions could be answered from readily available digital clinical reference sources. Chambliss[13] states that over half of unanswered questions by family physicians could be answered using MEDLINE™ and textbooks. Research by the PrimeAnswers Project[14] concluded that the critical factors in lack of use of digital sources among urban primary care providers were lack of time and lack of skill in articulating a particular question in the best source for the clinical answer.

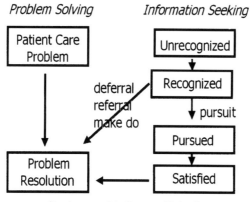

Based on research by Gorman and Osheroff

FIGURE 8.1. Context of information-seeking behavior.

$$\text{Usefulness of medical information} = \frac{\text{Relevance x Validity}}{\text{Work to access}}$$

FIGURE 8.2. Value of pursuing information.

Figure 8.2 is Shaughnessy's[15] equation for this work/value problem. He defines relevance as the frequency of exposure to the problem being addressed and the type of evidence being presented, the validity as the likelihood of the information being true, and work as the time and effort that must be spent extracting the information. The bottom line is that busy primary care providers sacrifice quality in deference to time. The ideal information source would be synthesized, brief and only an arm's length away.

Types of Questions and Answers

Much of primary care can be attributed to a limited number of complaints, and many decision tasks are routine or recurring[9,11,16]. A study of rural family practitioners in Iowa[11] found that questions about drug prescribing, obstetrics and gynecology, and adult infectious disease were most common and made up 36% of all questions. An expanded study[16] determined that the five most common types of generic questions, 27% of the total, were about drug of choice for a condition, cause for a symptom, test indicated for a situation, dose for a drug, and treatment for a condition. The largest number of questions related to drugs and other treatments for conditions.

Using contextual inquiry methods, the PrimeAnswers Project[14] found that the information resources most commonly used and desired by urban primary care provider's in an academic setting clustered into four categories: drugs and natural products; immunizations; travel medicine; and skin conditions. The types of materials used or desired were patient education; guidelines; textbooks to answer questions on diagnosis, therapy, and prognosis for uncommon presentations or conditions; primary literature; and consultation with colleagues. The participating physicians indicated that they would be most likely to use digital sources when a colleague was not available or in lieu of requesting a consult from a centralized service.

Based on this research, the most effective approach for answering the clinical questions about diagnosis, therapy, and prognosis is to begin with a predigested summary of the evidence. However, the provider also needs to look up fact-based information (e.g., recommended drug dosage, dermatology images to verify a condition). The optimal information source to answer a specific patient question depends, to a large extent, on the type of question and the time available. In the next section, we look at types of questions and illustrate specific sources to answer the questions that arose during our primary care providers morning clinic at the beginning of this chapter.

Questions about Drugs and Natural Products

The most common questions arising at the point of care are about drugs, particularly choice, costs, effectiveness, and potential harm. Popular drug handbooks with extensive information about effectiveness, interactions, and potential harm are available online (see Table 8.1) through a variety of vendors and formats. Many free drug sources of high quality are available on the Web for consumers and providers. Online information is updated more frequently than print handbooks and are searchable or can be browsed by class, category, or disease using simple navigation or search engines. Free sources may require registration and are often heavily subsidized by advertising. Proprietary drug information is also embedded in many physician order entry systems, electronic medical records, and other integrated reference textbooks and systems. Micromedex and eFacts are examples of an integrated drug reference systems. Beyond dose, cost, and interactions, such sources may provide pill identification, drug alerts, new drugs on the market, information on herbals and dietary supplements, patient education handouts, and poisoning and toxicological data.

Many providers routinely use a pocket drug reference (e.g., *Pocket Pharmacopoeia, Sanford's Antimicrobial Therapy*) to answer dose, cost, and antimicrobial questions. Applications for hand-held devices (see Table 8.2) are beginning to replace the traditional pocket paperback.[17,18] ePocrates capitalizes on the need for current, compact information on drugs (qRx) and antimicrobials (qID). Beyond a paper pocket guide, it provides automatic updates, integrated formularies, and provision for personal notes. New regulatory recommendations to reduce medication errors by eliminating handwritten prescriptions have encouraged a competitive marketplace for new technology products that combine electronic prescription services across multiple health plans with a traditional drug information source. To round out a digital pocket assistant, a provider might add a compact reference such as Griffiths' *5-Minute Clinical Consult,* some clinical calculators (e.g., severity indexes, predictive risk), immunization schedules, and local information such as a list of consultants. Digital pocket guides tend to be most popular among providers who do not have drug information integrated into their electronic medical record system and trainees moving between clinics.

Sources of evidence about the safety and effectiveness of herbals and natural products are rapidly becoming part of integrated on-line reference systems (e.g., AltMedDex in Micromedex). Natural Medicines Comprehensive Database, from the editors of *Prescriber's Letter,* exemplifies a new breed of predigested summaries of evidence targeted for use at the point of care. The data is formatted in tables covering interactions with drugs, diseases, lab tests, foods, and other herbal products as well as active ingredients, uses, dosing, mechanisms of action, safety, effectiveness, active ingredients, adverse reactions, and interactions and influence on nutrient levels.

Natural Medicines is the best source to answer our busy primary care provider's question about use of Ma-huang for weight loss and its effects in a diabetic teenage

TABLE 8.1 Sources of information about drugs, herbals and dietary supplements.

Source	Highlights	Availability	Cost*
AHFS Drug Information	American Hospital Formulary Service drug monographs	In: Medscape, STAT!Ref	Free, $
Clinical Pharmacology	Prescription, OTC, herbal and dietary supplements monographs with pill identification; patient education and medication profiling	www.cp.gsm.com Also in: WebMD	$$$
DRUGFACTS.com	Web portal linking selected drug information from Wolters Kluwer publications, headline news and drug tools for the public; professional content requires subscription	www.drugfacts.com	Some free
eFacts	Drug Facts & Comparisons, Drug Interaction Facts, Review of Natural Products, MedFacts for patients, Manufacturer Index, Drug Product ID	www.factsandcomparisons.com	$$$
FirstDataBank National Drug Data File	Drug database used primarily by hospitals and health plans	In: Medscape	Free
Medical Letter on Drug Therapeutics	Newsletter that critically evaluates new drugs	www.medicalletter.com Also in: SKOLAR, STAT!Ref	$
Micromedex Healthcare Series	PDR, DrugDex, AltMedDex, Martindale, USP DI for Professionals and Patients, PoisIndex, EmergIndex, Material Safety Data Sheets, hazardous management, reproductive risk, investigational drugs and dosing tools	www.micromedex.com Some patient information also in: familydoctor.org, MEDLINEplus	$$$
Mosby's GenRx	Monographs on prescription drugs	www.genrx.com Also in: MDConsult, STAT!Ref	$$
Natural Medicines Comprehensive Database	Summarized evidence on the safety, effectiveness and interactions of herbals and dietary supplements	www.naturaldatabase.com Also in: SKOLAR	$$
PDR.net	PDR suite of information on prescriptions and OTCs, herbals, interactions, patient education; news and advertising	www.pdr.net PDR also in: Micromedex	Free
USP Drug Information for Health Professionals	Monographs on prescription and OTC drugs, dietary supplements	In: STAT!Ref	$
USP DI Advice for Patients	Patient handouts on prescription drugs, herbals and dietary supplements	In: familydoctor.org, MEDLINEplus Also in: Micromedex	Free

*Cost per single user: $ < 100, $$ = 100–249, $$$ > $250

patient. Our provider searches for "ma huang" and retrieves a tabularized summary about ephedra, the generic name. Under the heading "Interactions with diseases and conditions," our provider reads that this substance many interfere with blood sugar control and may exacerbate high blood pressure and circulatory problems in people with diabetes. Performing the same search in AltMedDex leads to an ex-

TABLE 8.2 Digital pocket sources.

Source	Highlights	Handheld devices	Download address	Cost*
ePocrates qRx	Drugs, interactions, formularies, personal notes	Palm	www.epocrates.com	Free
ePocrates qID	Antimicrobials	Palm	ww.epocrates.com	Free
Tarascon ePharmacopeia	Drugs	Palm	www.medscape.com	Free
Adverse Drug Interactions	Handbook of Adverse Drug Interactions	Palm	www.medicalletter.com	$
Medical Calculator	Common equations for primary care	Palm	www.medscape.com	Free
MedRules	Clinical prediction rules	Palm	pbrain.hypermart.net/medrules.html	Free
Pocket Clinical Library	Several popular pocket-sized texts	Palm PocketPC	www.handheldmed.com	$–$$

For more programs see: pdamd.com or pbrain.hypermart.net
*Cost per single user: $ < 100, $$ = 100–249, $$$ > $250

tensive evaluation of the literature on Ma-haung, with diabetes listed as the first contraindication. Our provider contacts her teenage patient to ensure that she has discontinued use of this product.

Questions about Immunizations and Travel Medicine

The Centers for Disease Control and Prevention (CDC) provides a definitive and easy to use on-line handbook about immunizations and precautions needed for travel outside the United States (Table 8.3.) Updated schedules for adult and child immunizations and vaccination information are available in portable document format (PDF) to print as patient handouts. The questions generated by our busy primary care provider's second patient are easily formulated and answered using the CDC website.

Should you recommend a hepatitis A vaccination for a woman completing adjuvant chemotherapy for stage 2 breast cancer who will be traveling to Belize for a week's vacation? What is your recommendation for preventive treatment of travelers' diarrhea? Our provider links to Travelers' Health and finds "Health Information for Travelers to Mexico and Central America." A map indicates that Belize and all Central America are at high risk for hepatitis A. A deeper link recommends hepatitis A vaccine as safe for immunocompromised patients. For the question about traveler's diarrhea, she links to the "Food and Water Precautions and Travelers' Diarrhea Prevention" section on the CDC site, where it states that travelers are advised to "pay meticulous attention to choice of food and beverage" to help prevent travelers' diarrhea. However, the CDC does not recommend the prophylactic use of antibiotics even for immunocompromised travelers because antibiotics may cause additional problems.

TABLE 8.3 Specialized sources and textbooks.

Source	Highlights	Web address	Cost*
CancerNet	National Cancer Institute Information	cancernet.ncl.nih.gov	Free
Clinical Trials	Database of current clinical trials	www.clinicaltrials.gov	Free
ClineGuide	Textbook of specific recommendations on disease management and drug treatment	www.clineanswers.com or www.ovid.com	$$$
Dermatology Atlas Online	Database of more than 4000 color images with descriptions and differential diagnosis	www.dermis.net	Free
EthnoMed	Cultural issues in medicine	healthlinks.washington.edu/clinical/ethnomed	Free
GeneClinics	Disease-specific information on molecular genetic testing and its role in diagnosis and counseling	www.geneclinics.org	Free
Gene Tests	Directory of genetics testing laboratories in the U.S.	www.genetests.org	Free
Harrison's Online	Enhanced online version	www.harrisonsonline.com Also in: MerckMedicus	$
PubMed MEDLINE	Comprehensive index of biomedical journals from the National Library of Medicine	www.pubmed.gov	Free
Scientific American Medicine	Enhanced online version	www.samed.com Also in: WebMD	$$
Travelers' Health	CDC immunization recommendations and precautions for travel outside the U.S.	www.cdc.gov/travel	Free

Note: Many other textbooks are bundled on Web portals or by content aggregators. Journal tracking options include BioMail (biomail.org) or PubCrawler (pubcrawler.ie) for PubMed MEDLINE profiling, JournalWatch (jwatch.org), or journal briefs on portal sites. See Table 8.5 for a list of popular health portals.
*Cost per single user: $ < 100, $$ = 100–249, $$$ > $250

Questions about Skin Conditions

Another common need in primary care is information about abnormal skin or nail presentations. The need for diagnostic identification and an initial therapeutic approach with the patient in the office is required even when such patients are referred to dermatologists.

How would our primary care provider follow up on her 74-year-old patient with erythematous papules? An all-too-common scenario is that the clinic's dermatology textbook is missing or doesn't contain sufficient color images to match the patient's presentation. An electronic alternative called Dermatology Atlas Online is available on the Web (see Table 8.3). This atlas contains thousands of abnormal skin images. Our provider searches for "herpes zoster" and retrieves 17 images that denote the natural history of shingles. Using the zoom image feature, she decides that several images match the appearance and distribution of this patient's erythematous papules. With an initial diagnosis in mind, she links to UpToDate or Habif's *Clinical Dermatology* in MD Consult and finds a good description of the pathogenesis, natural history, and complications of shingles in an immunocompetent patient.

Questions about Best Evidence for Common and Uncommon Conditions

A new breed of evidence-based textbooks and high-quality systematic reviews are now available to answer questions about diagnosis, therapy, and prognosis of conditions relevant to primary care. There are two types of sources: (1) those that summarize evidence (e.g., *Clinical Evidence*) and (2) those that aggregate evidence sources (e.g., Evidence-based Medicine Reviews). Table 8.4 summarizes a selection of the growing field of evidence sources. In this section, we focus on six of them.

- The *Cochrane Database of Systematic Reviews* provides comprehensive coverage of a selected number of topics as a gold standard for best evidence on the effects of healthcare interventions through an international, nonprofit organization of centers called the Cochrane Collaboration. Each Cochrane review outlines the significance of the question being investigated, chronicles the extensive literature search undertaken and the methods used to analyze the results, summarizes the evidence in the best studies and contains recommendations for practice in a standard format. While Cochrane is considered the gold standard for best evidence, the number of reviews focused on questions relevant to primary care is relatively small. A predigested source such as *Clinical Evidence* that summarizes the results of Cochrane reviews is a better information-seeking approach for primary care providers.
- *Clinical Evidence,* a product of BMJ Publishing, summarizes randomized controlled trials and systematic reviews for relevance with an emphasis on the types of questions that arise in primary care care. Updated every 6 months, it covers about 400 questions or conditions. Most of the data relate to therapeutics. Both benefits and harms are listed and the authors take pains to point out gaps in knowledge by indicating where evidence is lacking. Only the evidence is provided—no expert recommendation is included—based on the assumption that the decision to apply evidence to patient care rests with the clinician.
- *Bandolier* began as a newsletter summarizing new primary research articles, and has expanded to tackle controversial, emerging, and difficult but common questions facing primary care providers. The summaries are succinct (the word "bandolier" name signifies "bullets" of information) and provide a careful synthesis of what is currently known about the efficacy of a clinically relevant intervention.
- *UpToDate* is an on line textbook designed to provide practical clinical advice for primary care. Expert authors synthesize the latest evidence and give specific recommendations for diagnosis and treatment. It includes a drug reference, patient information, tables and images, MEDLINE™ abstracts, and provision for CME credit. Updated every 4 months, it challenges the traditional expert-authored textbook through a successful combination of currency, ease of use, clinical practicality, and interpretation of evidence.

TABLE 8.4 Sources of evidence.

Source	Highlights	Availability	Cost*
ACP Journal Club Best Evidence Evidence-Based Medicine	Review of new research articles relevant to practice in internal medicine from ACP-ASIM and BMJ	www.acponline.com www.evidence basedmedicine.com Also in: EBMR	$$ Some free
Bandolier	Review of new research articles and key questions for primary care	www.jr2.ox.ac.uk/bandolier	Free
Clinical Evidence	Summarized textbook of evidence for primary care from BMJ	www.clinicalevidence.com Also from: Ovid	$$
Cochrane Database of Systematic Reviews (CDSR)	Gold-standard systematic reviews of health interventions from the Cochrane Collaboration	In: Cochrane Library, EBMR, SKOLAR	
Cochrane Library	CDSR, DARE	www.updateusa.com	$$
Database of Abstracts of Reviews of Effectiveness (DARE)	High quality systematic reviews of health interventions	nhscrd.york.ac.uk Also in: Also in: Cochrane Library, EBMR	Free
Evidence-Based Medicine Reviews (EBMR)	Best Evidence, CDSR, DARE	www.ovid.com	$$$
MedicalInfoRetriever	Review of new research articles and key questions for family medicine (POEMs), abstracts of Cochrane reviews, prediction rules, prescribing information	www.medicalinforetriever.com Available for: Palm, PocketPC	$ Some free
National Guidelines Clearinghouse	Database of structured summaries of clinical practice guidelines with a side-by-side comparison feature from the Agency for Health Research Quality	www.guideline.gov Also in: SKOLAR	Free
PubMed MEDLINE Clinical Queries	Search PubMed for best research studies on therapy, diagnosis, etiology, prognosis	www.pubmed.gov	Free
TRIP Database	Indexes evidence-based documents and articles from premier journals	www.tripdatabase.com	Free
UpToDate	Topical textbook reviewing latest research and providing diagnostic and treatment recommendations based on clinical experience in internal medicine.	www.uptodate.com	$$$

*Cost per single user: $ < 100, $$ = 100–249, $$$ > $250

- The *TRIP database* indexes a variety of evidence sources focused on the effectiveness of healthcare interventions. While the indexing is limited and there is a strong focus on documents created in the United Kingdom, TRIP is a free, fast, first step in ascertaining whether an evidence review exists on a particular topic. Recently it has expanded to index articles in core clinical journals and other materials on the Web. Another finding tool available in many medical center libraries is Ovid's *Evidence Based Medicine Reviews,* which retrieves Cochrane

reviews, ACP Best Evidence summaries, DARE articles, or topics in Clinical Evidence.
- The *National Guideline Clearinghouse*™ is a database for locating and comparing clinical practice guidelines. Sponsored by the Agency for Healthcare Research and Quality in partnership with the American Medical Association and the American Association of Health Plans, it includes over 1000 structured summaries. Links to the full guideline is dependent on the original source. Not all guidelines are evidence-based or relevant to primary care. The database is likely to be used for decisions on standards of practice for a clinic rather than care for a specific patient. Practice parameters and guidelines may also be found in MD Consult or Harrison's Online or directly from a society, association, or agency.

None of the products covers the broad spectrum of questions that arise in primary care. If a condition or question is reviewed, the evidence may be too meager or too general to make a decision on a particular therapeutic course for a specific patient. Currently these standalone products are islands of proprietary information rather than an integrated system that provides the busy practitioner seamless access to the best available answers. Let's look at how our primary care provider could use one or more of these evidence sources to find answers to the patient care questions that arose during her morning clinic.

Is there evidence that prescribing an antiviral, a corticosteroid, or both to a 58-year-old man with left-sided Bell's palsy is better than watchful waiting? Our provider first searches the Cochrane Library and finds there are two protocols in progress but no completed reviews. She moves on to Clinical Evidence and finds a succinct description of the evidence on drug therapy for Bell's palsy. Specifically, it states that while the combination of steroids and acyclovir and steroids alone have been used, there is not yet adequate evidence to support drug therapy.

What about the 72-year-old woman patient with osteoarthritis of the knees? Our provider wants to do some research on "coxibs" and traditional NSAIDS for pain control and GI bleeding. A TRIP search on "cox inhibitors" identifies a Bandolier review entitled "Cox-2 Roundup." Another click and our provider is perusing the review's comparison of the efficacy and adverse effects of Cox-2 and NSAIDS in acute and chronic pain. Bandolier typically provides helpful comparative tables and practical advice for primary care. To update this review, our provider searches the PubMed Clinical Queries database for "cox AND osteoarthritis" and finds some review articles published after the Bandolier review.

Is there an evidence-based review of the risks and benefits for HRT? Our provider searches for "hrt" in UpToDate and retrieves the ERT–risk of breast cancer and the more general ERT–benefits and risks topic reviews, in addition to an extensive patient handout. If our provider has a PC in the exam room, she can discuss this summary of evidence during the visit and print relevant sections for the patient to take home.

What are the latest recommendations for preventive treatment of travelers' diarrhea? Our provider returns to this question at the end of the day, as more of her patients will be presenting in the next month before they travel to sunny vacation spots in Central and South America. She searches Clinical Evidence and finds that empirical treatment with antibiotics shortens illness duration in adults with diarrhea acquired overseas and scans the discussion about nondrug preventive interventions, antimalarial vaccines, and antimalarial interventions in children and pregnant women. Moving on to the Cochrane Library, she finds a systematic review that concludes that antibiotic treatment is effective in reducing the duration and severity of symptoms but carries the price of increased risk of side effects. She turns to the CDC Travel Health source and searches for the new drug malarone and the new the fact sheet for health providers noting the most adverse effects.

Other Sources of Primary Care Information

Journal Literature

Our provider rounds out her research on antimalarials by searching for the prevention of malaria in PubMed MEDLINE™ to scan the most current literature. In this instance, two recently published articles draw her eye: a *Lancet* article comparing two antimalarials and a *New England Journal of Medicine* review on advice for travelers for primary care. Because she or her library subscribes to on-line versions of these journals, she is able to link directly from the PubMed reference to the full article.

Because most journal literature is estimated to have low relevancy to clinical practice in addition to the work involved in synthesizing numerous articles,[4] searching the MEDLINE database directly is usually reserved as a tertiary strategy for finding clinical answers in primary care. It is effective for finding information on uncommon conditions or presentations and for locating the very latest studies. ACP Journal Club, Evidence-Based Medicine, and POEMs offer evidence reviews of the most clinically relevant articles appearing in a core set of journals (see Table 8.3). DARE abstracts systematic reviews; PubMed MEDLINE™, the premier biomedical literature database, is updated daily and provides a simple and effective search engine with links to a growing number of on line journal articles. PubMed Clinical Queries searches MEDLINE for clinically relevant, high-quality studies through objective filtering using category limits (therapy, diagnosis, etiology, prognosis) and emphasis (sensitivity and specificity). Effective methods for searching MEDLINE for the best clinical results are available elsewhere.[19,20]

Searching the Web

There are occasions when searching the Web directly may retrieve a specific item needed for practice management. For example, our provider uses the Ottawa ankle rules to determine when one may safely decide not to take an X ray in the case of an injury. A patient incident relating to a decision not to X ray has arisen, and our provider wants to obtain the original published guideline. She uses Google (www.google.com), a popular Web search engine, and types "ottawa ankle rules guideline." Luckily, the first item retrieved links to the full guideline as published by the Alberta Clinical Practice Guidelines Program. Primary care providers do not usually find answers to patient care questions by randomly searching the Web, but in some instances this strategy may be a good approach. Providers may also refer their patients to specific association (e.g., familydoctor.org) or condition sites such as those selected for inclusion in the National Library of Medicine's MEDLINEplus™.

Aggregated and Specialized Sources

To find answers to general or uncommon clinical questions, a book chapter or annual review article by an authoritative expert may be the best (or only) available source of information. Popular textbooks such as *Goroll's Primary Care Medicine, Scientific American Medicine,* and *Harrison's* are available on line, and the ability to search the index, keywords, full text of the chapters, images, and figures allows the provider to find a specific item quickly. Many on line textbooks are updated more frequently than their print counterparts and include unique enhancements such as practice guidelines, updated research, and evaluative references (see Tables 8.3, 8.5).

MD Consult's reference book search of 35 textbooks is likely to retrieve some information on uncommon findings or conditions that primary care providers encounter. There are several competing aggregators or integrators of clinical reference that combine an interesting mix of drug reference, clinical textbooks, evidence sources, decision support tools, MEDLINE, online journals, new literature scans, patient information or handouts, health news, continuing education, and conference highlights. Table 8.5 describes some of the most widely known clinical reference portals. Several are available at no cost but display advertising or require registration or subscription to the most valuable professional content. Pocket Clinician Library brings together a selection of "coat pocket" guides for handheld PC devices (see Table 8-2).

Trends for the Future

The ideal information toolkit for primary care remains elusive for the time-pressed primary care provider. Best available evidence predigested from primary literature for clinical relevance must be continually updated and integrated into the electronic patient record of the future to become part of the provider's workflow. However, it is unlikely that technology can adequately interpret the need for complex and diverse patient specific information. Seamlessly aggregated content of multiple sources with a simple search interface activated by voice recognition or based on data from the patient's record will be required to meet information

TABLE 8.5 Health portals or clinical reference aggregators.

Source	Highlights	Web address	Cost*
familydoctor.com	Patient information (drugs, dictionary, conditions) from American Academy of Family Practice; popular for primary care patient handouts	www.familydoctor.com	Free
MD Consult	Integrated search of 35 textbooks and drug reference, 50 journals, drug database, practice guidelines, news, journal scan, patient education	www.mdconsult.com	$$
MEDLINEplus	Integrated search of patient information (dictionary, encyclopedia, directories, drugs, conditions, headline news) and identification of patient handouts from associations and agencies and self-help groups; from the National Library of Medicine	www.medlineplus.gov	Free
Medscape	MEDLINE, AHFS/FirstDataBank drug reference, palm tool downloads, conference highlights, journal scans, dictionary, patient information, CME, advertising	www.medscape.com	Free
MerckMedicus	Drug reference, patient education, Merck Manual, Praxis.md, news, and dictionary are free access; MD Consult, DXplain, Harrison's, and Cecil's restricted to registration by state licensed practitioners; from Merck and Co.	www.merckmedicus.com	All free to state licensed practitioners
Ovid On Call	35 textbooks and drug reference, Evidence-Based Medicine Reviews, Clinical Evidence, DXplain, Cline-Guide, 60 journals, MEDLINE, other literature databases	www.ovid.com	$$$$ Institutional subscription
Praxismd.com	Textbook of medicine, clinical alerts, evidence answers, drug reference, patient information, PubMed, journal scan, news magazine	www.praxismd.com	$
Stanford SKOLAR MD	Integrated search of 12 textbooks and drug reference, Cochrane Reviews, Natural Medicines, practice guidelines, MEDLINE, 45 journals; earn CME credit	www.eskolar.com	$$
STAT!Ref	Integrated search of 35 textbooks and drug reference	www.statref.com	by title
WedMD	Scientific American Medicine, Clinical Pharmacology, MEDLINE, journal scan, conference highlights, patient education, CME, news, email, practice management	www.webmd.com	e-health business integrator
SumSearch	Integrated search of small selection of medical databases that are freely available on the Web by condition and clinical objective	sumsearch.uthscsa.edu	Free

*Cost per single user: $ < 100, $$ = 100–249, $$$ > $250

needs of primary care providers. Such systems must include a new array of clinically relevant information and be accessible from a variety of digital devices. For example, GeneClinics provides genetic testing and counseling information and EthnoMed provides information about cultural beliefs in healthcare (see Table 8.3).

Some medical centers create their own aggregation of best clinical content using a variety of sources selected for quality, accessibility, and local relevance. At the University of Washington, librarians and clinicians have collaborated to create the Care Provider Toolkit, which integrates clinical references into a Web-based electronic medical record.[21,22] The PrimeAnswers Project,[14,23] funded by the National Library of Medicine, is using contextual inquiry methods to design an evidence-based information system for primary care physicians. Initially, the result is a blend of Web portal and digital pocket reference tools organized according to the question types identified by the target user group (e.g., drugs and herbals, immunizations, travel, skin, guidelines, calculators, predigested therapeutic evidence).

The Family Practice Inquiries Network (FPIN) [24], a consortium based at the University of Missouri, is creating answers to real questions from family physicians. The FPIN Answers are brief, structured summaries that review the evidence from a specified list of sources, summarize what others recommend, and provide a clinical commentary. Answers are published monthly in the *Journal of Family Practice (JFP)*, and a more comprehensive database is planned. Other primary care journals began publishing applied evidence articles in 2001, such as the Clinical Practice series in *New England Journal of Medicine*, the Applied Evidence series in the *JFP*, and the Cochrane for Clinicians series in *American Family Physician*.

Both the PrimeAnswers and FPIN projects recognize the importance of the clinical librarian as a cost-effective reviewer and distributor of best available evidence in primary care. Davidoff and Florance[25] anticipate that a new type of health professional called an informationist will emerge in the future. The informationist will be a core member of the patient care team. Although it is unlikely that an informationist will be integrated into every primary care practice, it is cost effective to build information systems that integrate synthesized information and a curbside consult service available to multiple clinics as a "broadband" library of the future. Such a system will be designed through deeper contextual inquiry into information workflow in primary care clinics and utilize the most appropriate new technologies to reduce time and question formulation barriers.

References

1. Ely JW, Burch RJ, Vinson DC. The information needs of family physicians: case-specific clinical questions. *J Fam Pract* 1992 Sep;35(3):265–9.
2. Gorman PN. Information needs of physicians. *J Am Soc Inf Sci* 1995 Dec; 46(10):729–36.
3. Gorman PN, Helfand M. Information seeking in primary care: How physicians choose which clinical questions to pursue and which to leave unanswered. *Med Decis Making* 1995 Apr–Jun;15(2):113–9.

4. Lock S. Does editorial peer review work? *Ann Intern Med* 1994 Jul 1;121(1): 60–1.
5. The online health care revolution: How the Web helps Americans take better care of themselves. Pew Internet & American Life Project. Nov 26 2000. http://www.pewinternet.org/reports.toc.asp?Report=26
6. Summaries for patients in each online issue of *Annals of Internal Medicine*. For example, Postmenopausal hormone use and primary prevention of heart disease and stroke in healthy women. *Ann Intern Med* 2000 Dec 19;133(12): S60. http://www.annals.org/issues/v133n12/nts/200012190–00003.html
7. MEDLINEplus, National Library of Medicine. http://medlineplus.gov
8. McAlister FA, Straus SE, Guyatt GH, Haynes RB. Helping patients integrate research evidence. *JAMA* 2000 Nov 22;284(20):2594–5.
9. Fletcher RH, Fletcher SW. Evidence-based approach to the medical literature. *J Gen Intern Med* 1997 Apr;12(Suppl 2):S5–14.
10. Smith R. What clinical information do doctors need? *BMJ* 1996 Oct 26;313(7064):1062–8.
11. Ely JW, Osheroff JA, Ebell MH, et al. Analysis of questions asked by family doctors regarding patient care. *BMJ* 1999 Aug 7;319(7206):358–6.
12. Alper BS, et al. Just-in-time electronic database investigation, unpublished. E-mail: alperbahealth.missouri.edu
13. Chambliss ML, Conley J. Answering clinical questions. *J Fam Pract* 1996 Aug;43(2):140–4.
14. Ketchell DS, St. Anna L, Revere D. The PrimeAnswers Project, unpublished contextual design research, Nov 2000. E-mail: ketchell@u.washington.edu
15. Shaughnessy AF, Slawson DC, Bennett JH. Becoming an information master: A guidebook to the medical information jungle. *J Fam Pract* 1994 Nov;39(5):489–99.
16. Ely JW, Osheroff JA, Gorman PN, et al. A taxonomy of generic clinical questions: Classification study. *BMJ* 2000 Aug 12;321(7258):429–32.
17. Lynn LA, Bellini LM. Portable knowledge: a look inside white coat pockets. *Ann Intern Med* 1999 Feb;130(3):247–50.
18. Freudenheim M. Digital doctoring: The race is on to put a computer into every physician's hand. *The New York Times* (Late Edition, Final) 2001 Jan 8;Sec C, p.1, col 2. http://www.nytimes.com/2001/01/08/technology/08HAND.html
19. Safranek S, Dodson S. Strategies for finding evidence. In: Geyman JP, Deyo RA, Ramsey SD, eds. *Evidence-based clinical practice: concepts and approaches*. Boston: Butterworth-Heinemann, 2000.
20. Haynes RB, Wilczynski N, McKibbon KA, et al. Developing optimal search strategies for detecting clinically sound studies in MEDLINE. *J Am Med Inform Assoc* 1994 Nov–Dec;1(6):447–58.
21. Fuller SS, Ketchell DS, Tarczy-Hornoch P, Masuda D. Integrating knowledge resources at the point of care: Opportunities for librarians. *Bull Med Libr Assoc* 1999 Oct;87(4):393–403.
22. Tarczy-Hornoch P, Kwan-Gett TS, Fouche L, et al. Meeting clinician information needs by integrating access to the medical record and knowledge resources via the Web. *Proc AMIA Annu Fall Symp* 1997;809–13.

23. The PrimeAnswers Project. http://healthlinks.washington.edu/primeanswers
24. Family Practice Inquiries Network. http://www.fpin.org
25. Davidoff F, Florance V. The informationist: A new health profession? *Ann Intern Med* 2000 Jun 20;132(12):996–8.

Recommended Readings

Armstrong EC. The well-built clinical question: The key to finding the best evidence efficiently. *WMJ* 1999 Mar–Apr;98(2):25–28.

Brigl B, Ringleb P, Steiner T, et al. An integrated approach for a knowledge-based clinical workstation: Architecture and experience. *Methods Inf Med* 1998 Jan;37(1):16–25.

Dwyer C. Ideas and trends: Medical informatics and health care computing. *Ann Intern Med* 1999 Jan 19;130(2):170–2.

Ebell M. Information at the point of care: answering clinical questions. *J Am Board Fam Pract* 1999 May–Jun;12(3):225–35.

Geyman JP, Deyo RA, Ramsey SD. *Evidence-based clinical practice: Concepts and approaches.* Boston: Butterworth-Heinemann, 2000.

Glanville J, Haines M, Auston I. Finding information on clinical effectiveness. *BMJ* 1998 Jul 18;317(7152):200–3.

Hunt DL, Jaeschke R, McKibbon KA. Users' guides to the medical literature: XXI. Using electronic health information resources in evidence-based practice. *JAMA* 2000 Apr 12;283(14):1875–9.

McAlister FA, Straus SE, Guyatt GH, Haynes RB. Users' guides to the medical literature: XX. Integrating research evidence with the care of the individual patient. *JAMA* 2000 Jun 7;283(21):2829–36.

McKibbon KA, Richardson WS, Walker Dilks C. Finding answers to well-built clinical questions. *Evidence-Based Med* 1999 Nov–Dec;4(6):164–7.

Miser WF. Critical appraisal of the literature. *J Am Board Fam Pract* 1999 Jul–Aug;12(4):315–33.

Sackett DL, Straus S, Richardson S, et al. *Evidence-based Medicine: How to practise and Teach EBM.* 2nd ed. London: Churchill Livingston, 2000.

Slawson DC, Shaughnessy AF. Obtaining useful information from expert based sources. *BMJ* 1997 Mar 29;314(7085):947–9.

Westberg EE, Miller RA. The basis for using the Internet to support the information needs of primary care. *J Am Med Inform Assoc* 1999 Jan–Feb;6(1):6–25.

9
Computer-Based Patient Education Resources and Instruction

CEZANNE GARCIA, M.P.H., C.H.E.S.

Scenario

A new adult patient calls to schedule a first-time appointment for a physical exam. A "new patient" packet is mailed and includes descriptive and contact information about the clinic and care team, including the clinic's Web site, a suggested preview of three health Web sites, and a patient-clinician e-mail address for questions and inquiries. Two days before the patient's visit, a reminder call about the date and time of the appointment is communicated via an interactive voice response system.

At check-in time the patient is welcomed by name by the desk staff, registration verification processing is completed, and the patient is given a decision-aid tool to write down questions that she wants to ask her doctor. She is asked to complete a medical history interview by computer in a private kiosk station in the waiting room. The computerized health history includes health status, health risk behaviors (smoking, exercise, and so on), and a checklist identifying her learning preferences and unique communication assistance needs. The information is entered into the patient's electronic medical record, and the health risk appraisal and learning preference information are immediately available for clinician review. Profiled is the patient's history of heart disease and her risk status of being a 10-year smoker. At the conclusion of the clinic visit, the patient is asked to return in two weeks for a follow-up appointment for her new diagnosis of hypertension and to further discuss her smoking. The nurse prints out a handout on hypertension, including three cardiac health information Web sites, and customized with the patient's name, smoking history, and care team members' names. The nurse briefly reviews how to screen for credible sites on the Web and encourages the patient to write down questions and bring in any questionable information she might find. The patient's ability to identify resources and briefly describe hypertension management is documented.

A week after her visit, the patient receives a computer-generated follow-up letter with health promotion tips tailored to her smoking behaviors and age-specific risk characteristics. At the next appointment, the patient arrives about 15 minutes early and notices a patient education kiosk in the waiting room. She clicks on a healthy heart video that helps her, through pictures and narrative, better understand the impact of her smoking on her high blood pressure. During her appointment the patient expresses her interest in trying to stop smoking and she is asked to view a computerized smoking cessation decision support tool using a private computer kiosk, the summary data of which profiles her stage of readiness to change her smoking behavior. She returns to the exam room where key points are reviewed and her questions are answered by her doctor. She expresses interest in finding out more about nicotine substitutes; smoking cessation support groups and behavior change options are discussed. A tailored education tool profiling the names of three support groups, one at the local community center and two on line, is given to the patient. A prescription for nicotine-laced gum is e-mailed to the pharmacy in her neighborhood. Later that evening, the patient e-mails the clinic with a question about using the nicotine gum right before meals.

Introduction

Patient education has emerged as an essential part of clinical practice as demonstrated by its position in accreditation criteria, various federal and state regulations, evidence-based practice guidelines and critical pathways, and state nurse and pharmacist practice acts. Additionally, health education interventions are increasingly recognized by health care providers as routine components of clinical care.[1] Its inclusion as a central component of quality clinical care is further supported by the Joint Commission on Accreditation of Healthcare Organizations (JCAHO), Health Care Financing Agency (HCFA), and Healthy People 2010's national health goals, incorporating minimum standards for the provision of patient education services.

Improving patient satisfaction with patient education has become a strategic goal for many healthcare practices serving both as a customer service standard and in recognition of its positive influence on market share.[2] With patient education correlated with overall patient satisfaction,[3-5] investing in patient education makes good market sense. Patient satisfaction has also been found to positively correlate with patient compliance[6] and increases the likelihood that a patient will return to a given health care provider.[7-10] As healthcare resources continue to shrink, feedback from patients is critical to targeting resource allocation *and* quality improvement efforts where they matter most.[11]

With over 70% of all Americans insured through a managed care plan,[12] the capitation system has created positive incentives to teach patients self-care strategies, which have led to improvement in their appropriate use of healthcare services.[13] The National Committee for Quality Assurance (NCQA), the accrediting organization for managed care organizations, has patient/member education guidelines that address health promotion as well as policies that support and recognize member participation in their medical decision-making process.[14] Managed care has also catalyzed consumer/patient-directed health information gathering. This consumer-driven information gathering is tied to reduced confidence in medical service utilization decision making due to increased payer influence in the brokerage of health care services. Furthermore, reduced clinic visit lengths that do not always allow patients' main educational concerns to be addressed have fueled this trend.

Your healthcare practice can be a constructive partner in patient-centered information gathering through a variety of sources, most notably the Internet. Consumer/patient use of computers to gather health information, increasingly referred to as e-health, is not only demonstrated by increasing incidents of patients bringing computer printouts of information from a Web site to guide their inquiries with their clinician about their healthcare options but also by recent consumer surveys on technology trends. A 1996 consumer health informatics report issued in the U.S. General Accounting Office showed that the consumer demand for health information and shared decisions is substantial and growing.[15] In the United States, one half of the estimated 70 million active users of the Internet are using it to obtain health information or support.[16,17] Furthermore, the Internet health information–seeking population is growing nearly twice as fast as the Internet population at large.[18] This demand for on-line health-related services is addressed by an ever-growing volume of publicly and privately sponsored healthcare sites.[18] Consumer interest in sites is being measured and the number of consumers served by one such site, PubMed, a search tool for accessing medical citations, increased by 200% after the National Library of Medicine made it available free to the public in 1997.[19] Payers and providers in healthcare are shifting their service delivery models to respond to these consumer/patient interests. A survey of approximately 250 payers and providers working in managed care and provider-based healthcare organizations stated plans to nearly double their business-to-consumer transactions using Web-enabled applications with the goals of improving customer satisfaction, enhancing quality of care, and reducing healthcare costs.[20]

Computer-based patient education tools come in a varied and complex array of applications. The goal is to meet patient's desires to be informed and educated about their health and related healthcare choices and to support the goals of healthcare providers and payers to improve care and control costs. Computer-based resources are tools, and alone, they do not achieve these goals. Clinical team involvement to screen and guide selection of these tools based on their quality and suitability is essential to assist patients with maintaining healthy behaviors, acquiring knowledge and skills for managing acute and chronic conditions, and making decisions about treatment. Information in this chapter is presented to help clinical teams tap the promise of computerized patient education applications and make decisions about utilization of these applications; to yield organizational workflow efficiencies; to become knowledgeable about the types of applications available to support patients' learning; and to increase understanding of the evidence base of these applications to improve health outcomes and patient satisfaction. Computerized educational resource management systems and interactive health communication applications offer new approaches to information delivery and patient instruction, and their use is supported by a growing body of research and experience.

Strategic planning is necessary to determine computer information system priorities to improve the likelihood that its benefits are achieved; success can be assured only when the system meets users' needs and matches the way information flows in your organization.[21] There is a scarcity of operational models available to guide users in the practical aspects of system selection, design, and implementation. This chapter provides information to focus decision making regarding the use of interactive health communications applications in multidisciplinary primary healthcare settings.

Information System Infrastructure and Patient Education–Related Application Choices

Your clinic's current or proposed computer-based information system infrastructure will affect the range of computer-enabled patient education resource options your staff considers. Hardware and software capability and power, technical support and training, and computer terminal access in your exam rooms and care delivery areas will influence your choices. Increasingly, large practices of healthcare systems involving multiple practice sites and/or clinic affiliates are relying on institution-wide networks that offer users of heterogeneous computing environments access to standardized applications. Answers to the following questions about your computer information system will influence your decision to adopt and use information technology applications.

1. Does your practice have a computer environment capacity that supports the data transmission speed, bandwidth capability, computer-processing power, information storage capacity, and transmission necessary for the selected or to-be-developed application(s)?
2. Does your clinical team have basic knowledge or access to staff training that will support the computer literacy needed to both use and support the application(s)?
3. Has there been a clinic workflow analysis to ensure computer terminal and printer access and compatibility in your exam rooms or care delivery areas that will assure clinician access to the application?
4. If the application is targeted for patient use outside the clinic setting, do most of your patients have access either in their home or in public locations to Internet-linked computers and/or software that can support the application?

Administrative information technology options to manage patient education resources and services reviewed in this chapter include the following:

• Electronic medical record documentation of patient learning
• Educational resources/materials management software
• Educational material production

Information technology–based learning experiences and resource options available to support your patient education include the following:

• Health risk appraisals
• Computer-assisted instruction and decision support (health instruction, clinical symptom or treatment monitoring, computer-mediated communication with health care team)

• Health information and resources access
• On-line support groups

Your patient education goals and learning objectives, a clear understanding of your information technology system's capacity, and the evidence base for computerized patient education applications can guide your selection and use of commercial and custom-designed educational tools to meet your specific patient education needs.

Electronic Medical Record Documentation of Patient Learning

Implementation of a point-of-care computer system that allows for automated documentation offers an appealing alternative to the time-consuming and ineffective methods of managing manual documentation. Many accrediting groups, including the Joint Commission on Accreditation of Healthcare Organizations (JCAHO), are using medical record documentation of patient education as a standard for evidence of practice; if it is not documented, it did not happen. As presented in Chapter 2 (Electronic Medical Record), benefits include improved access and quality to patient data, easier review of information, and increased timeliness of data communications. The strongest evidence of benefits tied to implementation of computerized patient records is increased quality of documentation.[22-24]

Integrating patient education documentation into your electronic medical record creates the potential for quick reference and standardization of your teaching plans and builds capacity to examine aggregate data for evaluating outcomes linked to your team's patient teaching. To optimize the benefits of documenting patient education, your team needs to decide what information will be recorded in your patient education fields, typically based on a combination of external standards from JCAHO (Table 9.1) and internal care standards. Minimally your patient education documentation should include the following:

• An assessment of your patient (and/or caregiver's) ability and readiness to learn, with specific reference to special needs such as a need for an interpreter and unique physical or cognitive adaptations that will support communication
• A brief description of the education process:
  What was taught and Why
  How the teaching was provided
  Outcome of teaching using action verbs to describe how the patient or family showed their knowledge or behavior change related to your teaching
• Follow-up needs based on the extent to which your patient indicates understanding or skill change

Clear, specific learning outcomes representing your interdisciplinary team's teaching priorities can be coded to standardize learning outcomes, speed the doc-

TABLE 9.1 JCAHO topics for interdisciplinary patient education–related knowledge and skill documentation.

Assessment of readiness to learn
Understanding of the diagnosis
Preparations for treatment/procedure
Reason for treatment
Planned treatment
Care-at-home instructions
Pain and the importance of effective pain management
Administration and safe use of medication
Safe use of medical equipment
Avoidance of food and/or drug interactions
Proper diet
Rehabilitation exercises and techniques
Personal hygiene suggestions
Follow-up care plan and referral
Community resources to aid recovery

Source: Joint Commission on Accreditation of Healthcare Organizations. *2000 Automated Comprehensive Accreditation Manual for Hospitals.* JCAHO, Oakbrook Terrace, IL, 2000.

umentation process, and to link to a notes section for narrative details as needed to help others with understanding each patient's unique needs.

Patient Education Materials Distribution and Storage Systems

Reinforcing patient teaching with clear, easy-to-understand patient education materials has been shown to improve patients' learning,[25] with increased benefits shown by a growing research base that demonstrates even greater learning achieved with customized message tailoring to individual user or community profiles.[26] Patients and families may have difficulty remembering verbal instructions, and written materials can reinforce and enhance information presented by their healthcare provider.[27,28] Reductions in unnecessary medical visits[29–31] and telephone calls[32] have been attributed to the use of written patient education materials. Criteria to screen and select written materials for your patient education collection to support your patient teaching should be the same for computer-accessed materials and their off-line counterparts. Whether you are selecting individual or a database collection of materials, material content criteria to apply include the following:

• Content accurately reflects your standard of practice or is easily modified to match your practice.
• Reading level is appropriate for your patient population (see Table 9.2).
• Illustrations are simple and reinforce important content or skills steps.
• Gender, ethnicity, religious, and commercial biases are absent unless the teaching tool's objective is to instruct on the use of specialized, brand-name equipment or medication.

TABLE 9.2 Selecting a reading level target for your patient education materials.

With more than half of all Americans unable to read and understand health-related handouts given to them in a hospital or clinic,[86] screening materials for patient readability and clinical relevancy is essential. To reach the maximum number of patients, select a three- to four-grade reading level range to guide your patient education material selection. With approximately half of the U.S. adult population reading at a fifth-grade reading level or higher,[87] you can use the fifth- to eighth-grade range, as have most commercial patient education material publishers. If you know your patient populations' education demographics or screen your patients' reading level using the Wide-Range Achievement Test (WRAT3)[88] or Rapid Estimation of Adult Literacy in Medicine (REALM) Test,[89] you can target a reading level range for materials that matches your patients' reading abilities.

If your practice reviews a high volume of patient education materials or is part of a large healthcare system and record keeping of material reviews will prevent duplication of effort, a standardized review form, such as that used at the University of Washington Medical Center, shown in Figure 9.1, can improve the efficiency of your clinical team's patient education material review process. If you are reviewing a commercially produced collection of materials, select a small, diverse sample of individual education materials and evaluate each one to gauge the collection's appropriateness for your practice.

Depending on the size and scope of your practice, time spent collecting, selecting, stocking, and ordering patient education and information resources varies tremendously and can benefit from computerized management options. There are over a dozen commercial computerized general and specialty health material collection programs that deliver ready-to-use patient education materials.

Advances in computer informatics have improved the information storage and retrieval capacities of database management software. To demonstrate the range and variability of commercial patient education material management program features, profiles of four commercial vendors are provided in Table 9.3. A more comprehensive listing of patient education material management software can be found at http://www.ohsu.edu/women/judkinsd/software.htm. The emergence of new technologies and the maturation of the patient education evidence base ensures a continued evolution of product development and integration to support improved clinical efficiencies and patient education material excellence.

Defining what you want your educational material management program to do will greatly influence the type of programs your team will evaluate. Factors to guide your selection and/or development of a computerized patient education material collection and management system include the following:

• Does the scope of health topics in the collection closely match your practice's priority teaching topics and the perceived information needs of your patients?
• Does the collection of patient education materials meet the comprehensiveness and depth of content needed to support your practice's scope of care? What gaps in your patient education material collection will be closed by purchasing the scope of topics available in the database? Do you currently have a core semiorganized collection of patient education materials that adequately supports

Dear _____ ,

Would you please take a few moments to review and evaluate the attached education tool based on the following criteria:

🙢 Need   🙢 Applicability   🙢 Medical Accuracy   🙢 Appropriateness
🙢 Consistency with UWMC Policies and Procedures

Please return by _____ to the address below.
Your assistance is very much appreciated.

Title: _____   Subject: _____
Reading Level: _____   Language: _____

Reader Addressed: ❑ Child   ❑ Young Adult   ❑ Adult   ❑ Other

I have examined this brochure and think it meets the following criteria:

Yes	No	
❑	❑	Medically accurate and up-to-date
❑	❑	Adequate to cover the topic
❑	❑	Clearly written at an 8th grade level or lower, or the reading level is correct for the reader addressed
❑	❑	Well organized/presented: Sections signified with subtitles/headers, adequate white space
❑	❑	Culturally sensitive for reader addressed
❑	❑	Consistent with UWMC policies and practices
❑	❑	Free of stereotypes (racial, sexual, etc.)
❑	❑	Enhanced by appropriate illustrations/graphics
❑	❑	Does not duplicate education materials currently available at UWMC

Please check one:
❑ Recommend this patient/family education tool.

❑ Recommend with reservations. Please specify: _____

❑ DO NOT recommend this patient/family education tool. Please comment: _____

Reviewed by: _____ Date: _____

Department: _____ Mail Box: _____

Phone:_____

Please return to:

Name: _____ Department: _____ Mail Box: _____

Phone: _____

Thank you   © University of Washington Medical Center

FIGURE 9.1. Patient education material evaluation form.

your team's teaching needs? Or is yours a new practice just starting to build a patient education material collection?
• Are the materials easy to modify or adapt to match your practice's standards of care? Is there a staffing commitment to manage the needed customization of the patient instructions?

TABLE 9.3 Examples of commercial patient education management programs

Tool name	Topics	Features	Tailoring the tool to your content or patient
Clinical Reference System http://www.patienteducation.com/	Over 8000 ready-to-print tools, written at grades 4–8 level, with illustrations Adult health Behavioral health Cardiology Discharge instructions Eye Medication Pediatric Senior health Sports medicine Women's health	Updated once a year; Medication Advisor updated twice a year. Single user and wide-area network The Adult Health Advisor, Pediatric Advisor, and Women's Health Advisor files have been linked coding for ICD-9 and CPT classifications.	Insert patient, physician, and practice names Topic customization is for certain fields only (e.g., medication dosage)
Krames-on-Demand http://www.staywell.com/kod/	450 ready-to-print handouts plus 150 in Spanish written at grade 6 level, with illustrations Cardiovascular Diabetes ER/trauma Family practice Gastroenterology General surgery Gynecology Health promotion Maternal and child health Obstetrics Oncology Orthopedics Pediatrics Pre-op/Post-op Pulmonary Radiology Rehab Senior health Stroke Women's health	Updated once a year Single stand-alone computer or on a local area network	Patient's name, who to call with questions, and logo

Medifor, Inc. http://www.medifor.com	Over 675 ready-to-print tools, written at grades 4–6 level, with illustrations Cardiovascular Dermatology ENT Gastrointestinal Genitourinary Health maintenance Immune/Hematologic Metabolic/Endocrine Musculoskeletal Neurologic/psychiatric OB/GYN Respiratory	Combines patient education material distribution with option to link to electronic medical record Updated four times per year Single stand-alone computer or on a local area network	Editor feature allows for customized templates and addition of practice guidelines and tie-in of outside educational resources: can specify pamphlets, books, articles, videos, Web pages, and 800 numbers Any clinical user can make content changes to the defaults in an EduCare Template and save them
Micromedex Care Notes http://www.mdx.com/	6000 ready-to-print tools, all in English and Spanish, written at grades 6–8 level; no illustrations General injury, illness, and procedure overviews Preprocedure or presurgical information Inpatient diagnostic/treatment process Discharge care Long-term treatment of illnesses, injuries, procedures, and surgery DrugNotes Emergency department after-care documents	Updated four times per year Single users, networks, and intranets	Customize and save content using SaveNotes (allowed only for users with administrative and edit rights) Users with view-only rights can insert clinician, practice, patient, and caregiver names and individualized patient care information

TABLE 9.4 Factors that make materials easier to read and understand.

Reading level goal that is three grade levels lower than the average education level of your patient population OR fifth- to eighth-grade level
Use of active versus passive voice
Short, simple sentences, 12–15 words long
Sections signified with subtitles/headers; use of bullets, boldface type, and underlining to guide the reader through the text
Interactive text that builds in review
Paragraphs limited in content to one key point
All technical/medical terms defined the first time they are used in the document
Culturally sensitive text and graphics
Simple illustrations and/or graphics that reinforce specific skill-building steps or facilitate understanding of health issue
Use of white space, large font size (minimum 12 points, 14 points for older audiences)
Location for contact information, phone numbers, clinic and/or staff names to allow for follow-up

Source: Adapted from University of Washington Medical Center's *Easy Writer 2.0 How to Create Materials Your Patients Will Use*©.

• Are the teaching tools in the collection written to ease comprehension, meeting your team's criteria or most or all criteria in Table 9.4.?
• Will access to ready-to-print computer-generated handouts reduce the collection size or management costs associated with your paper-based patient education material collection?
• Do you and others in your practice have the computer literacy skills that will support the use of the program's functions? Is specialized training support needed and provided, through either instruction or self-directed training models?
• Can your clinic's computer environment support the program's intended performance?
• Check the marketplace stability of the producing company and ask for current customer references to determine whether your technical support needs will be addressed in a timely manner and minimize system downtime.
• Does the product have a one-time-cost feature or an annual network or per-user license fee structure? Are the technical support services and training included in the fees?
• Are procedures for updating, removal, and the addition of new tools in the collection clearly stated?
• Who is involved with the development of materials distributed by the program? Are reputable health experts acquainted with clinical care and health education standards on the review board?
• Are you looking for a program that will support organizing and providing access to your materials at one or more sites?

Patient education material utilization patterns in clinical practice settings are poorly understood. Collections can become unyieldingly large and difficult to manage, especially if there are no clear material quality standards, limits to the scope of topics that your collection will support, and determined levels of tolerated redundancy. An observational study of 57 family medicine physicians[33] challenges trends toward the use of large communal libraries of patient education materials. Observations of physicians who used materials that were from large communal libraries showed that they were significantly less likely to use them to support their teaching, when compared to physicians who utilized small "personal stash" collections. Physician familiarity with available handouts and the ease of locating the ones they wanted to use were presented as key explanations for the observed use patterns. Your practice's educators and therefore primary patient education material distributors, whether they are physicians, nurses, or other healthcare providers, need to be actively involved in the materials selection process to assure that content meets their teaching needs and your patients' learning needs. Clinician involvement in selecting a collection will build staff knowledge of the content and increase the likelihood of the material's usefulness in everyday teaching encounters.

Developing a Patient Education Instructional Program

There are a variety of instructional authoring systems available on the market to help individuals with limited programming expertise apply cognitive and behavior concepts to create text and graphic displays for moderately complex Web and on-line learning applications. Psychosocial theory and models are frequently used by developers in selecting appropriate content, media, and methods, and knowledge of these theories can help with critically appraising the true value of these applications. Psychosocial concepts or theories that are particularly important in interactive health communication application development are empowerment,[33] self-efficacy,[34] and motivation.[35] Behavior change concepts integrated into computer-based applications to influence individual behavior include the following:

• Understanding of intended user motivation for change
• User belief that a proposed change addresses needs
• Social support
• Skills and self-efficacy
• Simple, easy-to-use implementation plans
• Pilot testing to allow for users to fail safely and learn in the process
• Monitoring and feedback[36]

Lesson options include drills, tutorials, simulations, and games with features to tailor an interaction to the specific needs of the individual user. Question structures can be multiple choice, yes or no, fill in the blank, matching, or word responses. Most applications involve record keeping for individual and/or aggregate data storage, analysis, and two-directional flow of information, or interactions between the computer and user. Clinicians considering application development should carefully weigh the typically high resource investment costs of application conceptualization, design, implementation, evaluation, and refinement activities.[36] Knowledge about behavior change concepts and theories can also be applied to help select and utilize commercially produced applications to support your patients' learning and behavior changes.

Computer-Based Applications That Support Patient Education, Health Promotion, and Informed Decision Making

The rapid growth in new technologies has yielded a wide range of computer-based applications that support patient education, health promotion, and informed decision making: computerized health risk appraisals, computer-assisted instruction and decision-making applications, Web-based information resources, and on-line support groups. To optimize learning, these applications increasingly are integrating adult learning and behavior change theories into interactive information, education, and support applications tailored to group and/or individual needs and preferences. Although many interactive health communication applications focus exclusively on one function, the newer generations of applications combine numerous functions (Table 9.5).

With technological advances in computer-based instruction evolving faster than theory and assessment tools, the *Report on Interactive Health Communication* was released by the Science Panel on Interactive Communication and Health in 1999 to provide guidance in application utilization, evaluation, and development.

From research completed in the 1980s and 1990s, we know that patients gain knowledge, learn skills, and can change health-related behaviors using videos and computer-assisted instruction at least as well as they can from one-on-one encounters.[37-42] A literature review completed by Lewis[43] on interactive computer-based approaches to patient education (most are interactive video or CD-ROM programs) supports computer-based patient education as an effective, easy-to-use strategy for transferring knowledge and skill development that is popular with patients. However, few controlled and comparative studies exist on the effectiveness of tools intended to empower patients to make informed medical choices and weigh the risks and benefits of treatment alternatives.[44] The 14-member nonfederal Science Panel on Interactive Communication and Health reached similar conclusions in its summary of the current evidence and science of the effectiveness of computer-based instruction applications and concluded that few interactive health communication applications have been adequately evaluated for quality or effectiveness.[36]

SCIPICH developed a purchaser's evaluation checklist http://www.health.gov /scipich for interactive health applications to help with the decision-making process:

1. Why was the application developed?
2. What does the program propose to do?
3. What are the technical requirements of the application?
4. Does the program work as described?
5. What are the probable benefits for my specific organization (why should senior management buy in)?

TABLE 9.5 Functions of interactive health communications.

Function	Definition	Examples
Relaying information[90,91]	Provide general or individualized health information on demand	Web sites On-line services Telephone-based applications that use interactive voice response and fax-back technology
Enabling informed decision making[44,59,92-97]	Facilitate the health decision-making process of individuals and/or communication between healthcare providers and individuals regarding the prevention, diagnosis, or management of a health condition	Assist users with healthcare decisions such as selecting a health care professional, health plan, or nursing home Assist users in evaluating and selecting options that are consistent with desired health outcomes
Promoting health behaviors[98-102]	Typically based on theories of behavior change; promote the adoption and maintenance of positive health behaviors on both an individual and community level	Risk assessment modules Health promotion modules
Promoting peer information exchange and emotional support[51,54,61,95,103-109]	Enable individuals with specific health conditions, needs, or perspectives to communicate with each other, share information, and provide and receive peer and emotional support	On-line support groups for almost any health condition or health-related need Participants include consumers, patients, health professionals, and family caregivers
Promoting self-care[100,109,110]	Help users manage health problems without direct intervention from a healthcare professional or supplemental existing health service by facilitating remote health monitoring and care	Computer-assisted instruction
Managing demand for health services[13,100,111-114]	Provide specific information, tools, and other resources to support wellness, self-care, and self-efficacy to enhance utilization of effective health services and reduce use of unnecessary services	Computer-assisted telephone advice systems Interactive voice response systems Clinician-patient e-mail Electronic consultations with health professionals

Source: Adapted from SCIPICH-defined functions.[36]

Health Risk Appraisals

Computerized health risk appraisals solicit user responses to a series of health-related questions and demographics and run the individualized information through risk algorithms; the resulting calculation yields a statement of prioritized health risks for the individual. These programs typically include suggestions for reducing risks, and additional features may include referrals to resources and programs that target the user's health promotion profile and a health status summary that includes a "health age." A small number of studies on computerized history taking and health risk interviewing have shown that some patients prefer to provide information about personally sensitive issues in this way;[45-47] some patients are more likely to be truthful to a computer.[48]

Despite the popularity of these tools among users, early generations of the products were flawed because their calculations were based on standardized health data that did not reflect the different user populations.[49] The quality and value of these products has been enhanced by improvements in the accuracy of the data sets and risk algorithms, the development of specialized applications focusing on unique health conditions, and the use of individual and aggregate data to determine follow-up service and program referrals that offer tailored messages with individualized specifications. Concerns about the use of these tools involve their misuse by employers or payors reviewing the personalized health risk data to influence insurance coverage or persuasively influencing health risk–reduction activities of the employee using techniques that infringe on employee choice and privacy. At the very least, these tools serve as good marketing tools that hold appeal for their target audience with modest health impact. The utilization of health appraisals to create tailored health promotion programs and links to patient charts for clinician reference and counseling holds promise of benefits that promote patients' health and well-being.

Computer-Assisted Instruction and Decision Support

The content and purpose of computer-assisted instruction for patients and healthcare consumers range from tutorials that enhance knowledge and/or skills related to self-care to health-monitoring systems. These tools come in an array of formats including CD-ROM, Web-based, and Internet platforms. Computer assisted instruction and decision support products can function as follows:

- Give information including reference information (integrated collection of patient information/education resources that may include general health and fitness magazines, reference books, pamphlets, encyclopedias, medical dictionaries, and/or certain medical and professional periodicals)
- Explicitly teach a targeted health topic
- Teach informed consent and/or effective informed decision making
- Teach how to perform a procedure and provide social and emotional skill training
- Encourage self-triage or be combined with automated triage with personal contact

CD-ROM and Web-based products are typically restricted to an individual computer or a computer network. Currently, CD-ROM and Web-enabled products have the marketplace lead on customizing content and creating individually tailored education printout features. Recent generations of CD-ROM products and their newer Web-based counterparts have increasing graphic sophistication of on-screen displays and customization features for printouts. However, this increased graphic sophistication requires the viewing terminals to have extensive hardware and software capabilities to support the program. The average home computer environment should be used to define the level of graphic and sound sophistication required for Web-based products your practice sponsors to ensure your patients' usability of the displays and printouts.

The more elaborate CD-ROM products that are intended for use in your clinic setting require clinic investment in expensive hardware that can support color print and video media, as well as provide the level of graphic and sound fidelity to optimize program utilization. Computer-assisted instruction can offer the following advantages:

• Just-in-time availability
• Private learning environments
• Programming algorithms that allow individualization of information presented
• Ability to simulate life experiences
• Immediate reinforcement of the learning
• Support for the decision-making process

Patient data entry for electronic diaries has primarily used conventional personal computer keyboards, touch screens, or even voice-activated entry. Newer applications feature remote handheld personal device assistants (PDAs) and may not require more than a phone line hookup for clinical team communication. With patients typically arriving at their doctor appointment 15 minutes early and average waiting room times of 22 minutes,[50] a selectively programmed computer for patients in your waiting room with interactive health instruction programs and/or access to computerized patient information databases and health resources could encourage patient-directed learning and information gathering during this waiting time. "The challenge for health professionals and purchasers is to identify systems that are effective and warrant further investment of resources, time and integration into clinical practice and preventive programs."[36]

Newer, evolving computer-assisted patient education instruction modules are increasingly integrating the use of algorithms that apply individual user demographics and responses to questions and create tailored education messages and activities. These applications may contain one or more features including knowledge or skill-building instruction, self-care decision making, electronic patient care diaries, and links to peer patient groups or clinician e-mail communication. Individual- and community-tailored health messages have been shown to be effective in improving awareness and knowledge changes in a variety of healthcare and promotion-related topics.[26] However most information technology–based applications have not been adequately studied to ascertain their impact on clinical outcomes, cost effectiveness, or clinician and patient satisfaction.

TABLE 9.6 Some heavily visited health-related newsgroups.

alt.fertility
alt.med.cfs.
alt.support.anxiety-panic
alt.support.arthritis
alt.support.asthma
alt.support.crohns-colitis
alt.support.depression
alt.support.diet
alt.support.headaches.migraine
alt.support.mult-sclerosis
alt.support.stop-smoking
misc.health.diabetes
misc.kids.health
sci.med.aids
sci.med.diseases.cancer

Support Groups and Self-Help Communities On Line

The most commonly used and valued on-line consumer-based health resource is peer support groups featuring knowledgeable persons (defined as both clinicians and peers) responding to patients' questions.[51] These electronic support networks are run predominantly by and for informed, committed volunteers. The users of on-line support groups are seeking comfort and support of those addressing similar life challenges and health information, and they are collaborating with others to advocate new research, services, and directions in health policy.

There are thousands of groups available on the Internet with discussion forums or newsgroups (formerly known as members-only message boards), and listservs offer information and emotional support groups on a wide variety of topics; Table 9.6 shows a sample of the range of topics of some heavily visited health-related newsgroups. Commercial on-line support services maintain subscriber-only message boards or support groups, which require subscribers to view messages posted on virtual bulletin boards. Listservs or mailing lists are similar to newsgroups, but messages are posted directly to subscribers' e-mail addresses and are typically unmoderated. Directories of on-line support groups are available at google (http://groups .google.com/googlegroups/deja_announcement.html) or Dictionary.com (http:// www.dictionary.com) or Topica (http://www.liszt.com). Archived recent postings to a newsgroup site's FAQ (frequently asked questions) sections can help gauge the group's personality and determine whether the topics discussed match users' interests or needs. Klemm and colleagues[52] built a framework to categorize messages of on-line support groups according to the following eight subject areas:

• Information giving/information seeking (questions and answers about diagnosis, treatment, medications, resources, and research)

- Encouragement/support (expressions of understanding and experience)
- Personal experiences (hands-on knowledge about the caregiving experience)
- Personal opinion (individual statements of personal belief—usually begin with "I think," "I feel," or "It's my belief")
- Prayer (statements regarding spiritual intervention or "otherworldly" intercession)
- Thanks (usually in response to request for help or information)
- Humor (jokes, amusing stories, personal anecdotes)
- Miscellaneous (list housekeeping duties and off-topic posts)

A review of several studies on the content and relevance of on-line support groups for specific conditions shows that actual content of on-line discussions varies considerably depending on the nature of the disorder and composition of the group.[53-57] Alemi and coworkers[58] compared voice-based electronic support groups with face-to-face support groups and found that the on-line groups over time were eight times more likely to meet than other groups. The electronic support group participants were also found to be less likely to visit a healthcare provider without an adverse impact on health status, suggesting that electronic support groups may help reduce inappropriate use of health services. In a randomized control study of HIV-infected patients that examined an interactive health communication application with multiple functions, encouragement/social support was the most frequently used function of the application. The study also showed that patients with access to the application were more likely to report higher quality of life in several dimensions, including social support and cognitive functioning than were the controls.[59] The SCIPICH panel concluded that the importance of electronic support groups can lead to substantial reductions in use of services and cost of care in certain groups.

On-line support groups can also help mediate some of the logistical barriers of traditional in-person support group attendance: problems of geography, time, physical disability, lack of respite care, and other constraints.[57, 60] While there are reports on the sharing of inaccurate and potentially dangerous medical advice in on-line groups,[61, 62] there are also reports of a self-correcting mechanism that deals with suggestions for unconventional and unproven treatments.[61] On-line support groups also represent a unique opportunity for clinicians to learn more about the needs of patients.

Internet Health Information and Resources

The Internet offers unprecedented access to health-related information and resources, with unique challenges and risks. The number of health-related Web sites is expanding (a current estimation is 15,000 to 20,000 health-related sites), and many sites are evolving with updates and design improvements. The ease and option of low-cost "publishing" on the Web creates an unparalleled environment for promoting and featuring a tremendous range of health-related information—and concomitant opportunities for misrepresentation. Although many studies have substantiated the inaccurate health information on the Web,[62, 63] many healthcare

TABLE 9.7 Guidelines for evaluating health information on the Web.

It should be clear who is providing the medical data; their qualifications should be posted.
Find out who owns the site and consider possible biases.
Make sure there is a way to contact the site owners. If you use the site and need to contact them, keep track to see if they respond in a timely manner.
Look for sites with recent postings; health information does get outdated.
If you have questions about something you find on the Web, ask your doctor or healthcare provider.
When you link to other locations on a Web site, check the Web site address to determine whether you have linked to a new site. There are tools available to help you more thoroughly evaluate Web sites such as http://healthlinks.washington.edu/help/navigating/#three or http://www.discern.org.uk.

resources on the Internet are reputable. The concern of possible endangerment of patients by low-quality medical information has driven most of the studies investigating the quality of medical information on the Internet.[67] "Patients have always obtained information outside the formal healthcare system. Perhaps now there is simply a new carrier called the Internet, and nothing else has changed."[65] Studies have shown that access to health information can help patients be more active participants in their care and lead to better health outcomes,[66, 67] but the Internet has also enhanced the importance of substantiating the source and accuracy of health information. The Agency for Health Care Policy and Research, Mitretek Systems, and Health Information Technology Institute defined seven criteria for evaluating the quality of health information provided on the Internet:[68]

- *Credibility*   Includes the source, currency, relevance/utility, and editorial review process for the information
- *Content*   Must be accurate and complete, and an appropriate disclaimer must be provided
- *Disclosure*   Includes informing the user of the purpose of the site, as well as any profiling or collection of information associated with using the site
- *Links*   Evaluated according to selection, architecture, content, and back linkages
- *Design*   Encompasses accessibility, logical organization (navigability), and internal search capability
- *Interactivity*   Includes feedback mechanisms and means for exchange of information among users
- *Caveats*   Clarification of whether site function is to market products and services or is to provide information

There are different systems for applying these information quality controls to Internet sites, each with unique strengths and shortfalls.[64] Clinicians can help patients become discriminating and informed medical consumers of on-line information by providing simple guidelines to evaluate Web sites (Table 9.7).

Kim and colleagues[69] reviewed 29 studies featuring criteria used to evaluate health information on the Web and found a high level of agreement on key evaluative criteria. However, Kim's review concluded that there remains a need to de-

TABLE 9.8 Examples of WWW sites with teaching materials and health information referral services for patients/consumers (September 2000).

Site name/Purpose	Site address
New York Online Access to Health (NOAH)	http://www.noah-health.org/
Information from Your Family Doctor	http://familydoctor.org/
Clinical Trials Linking Patients to Medical Research	http://clinicaltrials.gov/
MEDLINEplus	http://medlineplus.nlm.nih.gov/medlineplus
Columbia Home Medical Guide	http://cpmcnet.columbia.edu/texts/guide/
Combined Health Information Database	http://chid.nih.gov/

fine and test the validity and credibility of a simple set of criteria that the general public can confidently use and easily apply.

Another option for confirming the credibility of Web sites is for clinicians to refer patients to indexes that rate medical Web sites[90] or to proposed filtering technologies that label valuable health information sites and dubious information sites.[64] However, a review of 47 proposals for Internet labeling standards for health information concluded that it was unclear "whether they measure what they claim to measure, or whether they lead to more harm than good."[71]

Examples of Internet sites dedicated to help clinicians and consumers/patients evaluate and screen out dubious medical advice and sites include OMNI (http://omni.ac.uk/), HON (http://www.hon.ch/HONcode/Conduct.html), Quackwatch (http://www.quackwatch.com/) and Discern (http://www.discern.org.uk/). A drawback to these sites is that they slow down the process of locating quality information, as each Web-based resource needs to be checked manually against a set of criteria.

With the growing number of health-related Web sites, search engines, kindred to on-line yellow pages, can be useful tools that enable users to quickly locate relevant information on user-selected topic(s). Most search engines feature a "help" section that provides guidance on how to best utilize the search engines, tips on how to improve prospects of finding relevant sites, and an overview section that defines the site's screening criteria. Some search engine sites also offer subdirectories or term-based searches of their site. Furthermore, some search engine sites, such as Healthfinder (http://www.healthfinder.gov./) and Health InfoQuest, pathfinders to common consumer health questions, (http://nnlm.gov/healthinfoquest/), focus solely on brokering links to health-related sites.

Most clinicians do not have the time to diligently and regularly monitor the emerging Web sites that potentially could benefit their patients and address their health concerns. Work with your health care team to identify three to five general and/or specialty health topics and feature only two to three Web sites per topic. Tables 9.8 and 9.9 give short lists of Web sites for a general health scope and for specific health topics.

Consider selecting "safe" sites, typically those sponsored by government agencies, professional medical organizations, and major national disease-specific organizations. These sites characteristically have strong advisory boards and credible sources and are updated regularly. The "thumbprint" letters in the last three

TABLE 9.9 Short Web site lists on select health topics

Cancer-related Web sites	Web site address	Brief description
CancerNet	http://cancernet.nci.nih.gov	Contains material for health professionals, patients, and the public, including information about cancer treatment, screening, prevention, supportive care, and clinical trials, and CANCERLIT, a bibliographic database
American Cancer Society	http://www.cancer.org/	Includes guidelines, publications and information (some full text) published or sanctioned by ACS. Click on icon for information about specific ACS programs.
Cancercare	http://www.cancercare.org	Includes online recorded teleconferences, information on specific cancers, and good material on fatigue and pain. Their on-line copy of *Helping Hand: The Resource Guide for People with Cancer* is searchable by geographic region, cancer site, and type of services offered.

Diabetes-related Web sites	Web site address	Brief description
American Diabetes Association	http://www.diabetes.org/	Offers an array of information resources
HealthAtoZ	The URL for the type 1 diabetes site is http://www.healthatoz.com/atoz/diabetes1/diabetesindex1.asp The URL for the type 2 diabetes site is http://www.healthatoz.com/atoz/diabetes2/diabetesindex2.asp	HealthAtoZ, a large consumer health site with diabetes information and resource listings

Multiple sclerosis-related Web sites	Web site address	Brief description
Multiple Sclerosis Foundation	http://www.msfacts.org/	Support service information on complementary and conventional healthcare options to address the varied symptoms associated with MS
National Multiple Sclerosis Society	http://www.nmss.org/	Local resources, education, and information tools and activities
National Institute of Neurological Disorders and Stroke Multiple Sclerosis Information Page	http://www.ninds.nih.gov/health_and_medical/disorders/multiple_sclerosis.htm	Defines multiple sclerosis, treatments, prognosis, and research

letters of organizations' Web addresses are a strong clue about the "domain" or sponsor of the site:

Government agency name.**gov**
Nonprofit professional medical organization's name.**org**
Nonprofit national disease-specific organization's name.**org**
Private company/product vendor name.**com**
Educational institution's name.**edu**
Internet service's name.**net**

A cautionary note: These Web site address thumbprints are not a substitute for closely scrutinizing the credentials of the site's information advisory board or authors and checking for the obvious signs of marketing goods or services. Furthermore, some sites sponsored and maintained by commercial or private individuals are both informative and valuable. In fact, medical searches completed by *Consumer Reports* for a story on getting medical help on line found that some of the best sites were maintained by private individuals.[72] But by recommending privately and/or commercially sponsored sites, your team needs to commit to continuously monitoring and reviewing the content of updates for accuracy and a sustained noncommercial focus.

More and more on-line sites are serving as portals or gateways to a series of related Web sites with interrelated information. Examples of directories of linked health Web sites that are available include the Hardin Meta Directory of Internet Health Sources (http://www.lib.uiowa.edu/hardin/md/index.html) and the healthcare provider resources site Medical Matrix (http://www.medmatrix.org/reg/login.asp). Strategies clinicians can use to improve on-line health information include educating their patients on how to independently evaluate Web site credibility, encouraging the use of self-imposed codes of conduct for Web masters (Health on the Net Foundation, HON), supporting independent consumer protection sites that monitor for and flag misleading and unsupported health claims (quackwatch.com, eHonor), and endorsing Federal Trade Commission and Food and Drug Administration regulation and law enforcement. Other new emerging strategies to improve on-line health information include Credential Search Service, which verifies physicians' credentials referenced in editorial boards and as Internet authors (http://www.tese.com/css/) and experimentations with subscriber-accessed services that use a physician review board to appraise Web sites' trustworthiness and electronically tags or labels these sites for subscribers.

When a patient comes to you with information from an Internet source, be positive:

• Welcome your patient's inquiries about health information from Web and other sources. Most Web site review criteria tell patients to consult with their healthcare provider and that no information found on the Internet should serve as a substitute for their healthcare provider's advice.[69]
• Encourage your patient's independent clarification of information through posting a query on a newsgroup or listserv.

• Encourage and help identify key words to run further searches at other sites or a journal article search on a high-quality refereed site, such as Medline (http://medlineplus.nlm.nih.gov/medlineplus/), to determine whether other sources support the information obtained from a Web site.

You can provide an alternative to the unlimited health information resources on the Internet by placing in your office a patient education kiosk with limited access to approved Web sites and/or to a commercial patient education reference database. Commercial patient education reference databases intended for direct patient/consumer use typically provide access to an integrated collection of patient information/education resources including general health and fitness magazines, reference books, pamphlets, and/or select medical and professional periodicals.

Impact of Technology-Based Patient Education on Clinician-Patient Communication

The volume and increased ease of access to health information is changing patient and consumer perceptions about authorities for health information.[36] Healthcare providers are becoming one of many sources of authoritative medical knowledge, shifting the balance from a clinician's role as an "authority" to a role as a "partner" with their patients. Although the important influence of the physician-patient relationship on patients' health outcomes is recognized,[73] our knowledge of how computer-based patient education strategies can be used to positively enhance patient-clinician communication is very limited.[36, 44] Ideally, clinician referral of patients to quality computer-assisted patient education instruction modules and information resources can supplement the information and support provided during a clinic visit and optimize limited time available for face-to-face patient teaching. Three studies profiled in a literature review[43] studying the effectiveness of computer-based education for transfer of knowledge and skill development for patients described these applications as supportive of the communication between patient and provider.[75–77]

Interactive health communication applications that specifically target the relay of information and manage the demand for health services include computer-assisted telephone advice systems, clinician-patient e-mail, electronic consultations with health professionals, and interactive voice response systems. Although consumer interest in these alternative approaches to communicating with doctors is growing, there currently are very limited opportunities for consumers to engage their doctors on line;[18] the benefits and impact of these approaches need further study. The conclusions of the literature addressing the impact of computer-based applications on clinician-patient communication is incomplete and presents conflicting conclusions. Keoun[78] discusses how information and advice from on-line information sources can be used to challenge clinicians, with the use of inappropriate applications leading to unnecessary conflicts and confrontations between consumers and their healthcare providers.[79] In contrast, Gustafsom and colleagues[59] showed that patients have increased confidence in their healthcare providers when they work with them to access and utilize interactive health communication applications. Borowitz and Wyatt,[80] in examining shared decision-making tools and provider-patient electronic communications applications, described improvements in the clinician-patient relationship. Clinician understanding of patient needs improved, and the delivery of reminders improved their communication with patients.

Costs

In spite of the promises by vendors and their customers of how computerized tools and Internet resources can cut overhead and administrative costs, financial models need to be developed and tested to help clinical practices manage and broker decision making on the cost effectiveness of patient education–related computerized products and office management tools.[36] Although better methods are needed for determining the impact of computer-based information systems on quality care at an affordable price,[81] this lack of cost-saving evidence is partly due to the difficulty in separating the effects of computer information systems and organizational change.[82]

Costs associated with computerized patient education system investments include capital investments for software and hardware, staff training for implementation and updates, technical computer support personnel, and operational costs that include supplies and, for some products, annual license fees. Implementation and maintenance costs associated with applications vary tremendously. There are no comparative studies of the cost and effectiveness of different informatics tools and decision aids on patient decisions about medical screening and treatment, especially for comparing and contrasting computerized versus noncomputerized ones.[44]

Some pragmatic suggestions to start you off:

1. Think about how your practice uses information, how you might use it differently, and how technology could support your current and potential uses. Recognize the human limits to capitalizing on these efficiencies.[81]
2. Familiarize your clinical team with the scope of available consumer and patient informatics tools. Some of the more sophisticated multimedia features may require prohibitively substantial capital to acquire or update equipment.
3. Define and focus on your patient population's learning style preferences for written, audiovisual, or interactive learning tools. Ask a sample of patients to write a letter to your practice describing their ideal patient communication and learning environment.
4. Specifically inquire about your patients' access and current use of computers. Although consumer trends inform us of increased computer use for health information, we also know that socioeconomic boundaries preclude technology access for some population groups.[83, 84] There currently are few initiatives to

improve access to technology for low-income populations, residents of rural areas, and people with disabilities.[36]

5. There is a nominal cost for creating a resource list of recommended Web sites and promoting guidelines to help your patients identify reputable sites and evaluate on-line health information and support groups. Physicians are looked to by their patients to guide and influence their health information uses; patients are more likely to look at materials recommended by their physicians[85] and prefer patient education resource recommendations of their physicians.[33]

6. Identify and support at least one staff member in your practice for building knowledge of computers and related computer applications and functions for the purpose of understanding potential uses and impact on your organization and health outcomes. Although healthcare lags behind other businesses in adoption of computer-based information systems,[89] this gap is closing as information systems are increasingly being applied to improve efficiencies and manage the large volume of health and administrative data used for clinical decision making and required by payors.

Conclusion

The rapid development of new technologies has created tremendous potential for improving clinical practice efficiencies and creating a supportive learning partnership between clinicians and their patients for optimizing health status. The scientific knowledge about many aspects of interactive health communication is very limited, but there is little doubt that these applications will grow in utility and popularity with clinicians and their patients who turn to them for health information, communication, and support. Whether your primary care practice is a small, independent clinic or integrated into a large healthcare system, careful evaluation and a systematic approach to decision making will help your organization determine how to best use administrative and interactive health communication technology to optimize your practice's efficiency. Ultimately, e-health tools can improve the ways clinicians work with their patients to prevent disease, maintain health, and support recovery from illness.

References

1. Center for the Advancement of Health. Health behavior change in managed care status report. Washington DC, 2000.
2. Crosson K, Nakamura RB, Simmons R. Health People 2010 Objectives for the Health Care Setting. Health Promotion Practice 1:3:243–244; 2000.
3. Findham JE, Wertheimer AI. Predictors of patient satisfaction in a health maintenance organization. Journal of Health Care Marketing 6:6–11, 1986.

4. Robbins JA, Bertakis KD, Helms LJ, Azari R, Callahan EJ, Creten DA. The influence of physician practice behaviors on patient satisfaction. Family Medicine 26:17–20, 1993.
5. Schauffler HH, Rodriguez T, Milstein A. Health education and patient satisfaction. The Journal of Family Practice, 42:1:62–68, 1996.
6. Haynes, RB. A Critical review of the 'determinants' of patient compliance with therapeutic regimens, in: D.L. Sackett and R. B. Haynes eds., Compliance with therapeutic regimens. Johns Hopkins University Press, Baltimore, MD, 26–39, 1976.
7. Marquis MS, Davies Ar, Ware JE. Patient satisfaction and change in medical care provider: a longitudinal study. Medical Care 21:821–30, 1983.
8. Herzlinger RE. The failed revolution in health care—the role of management. Harvard Business Review 99:95–103, 1989.
9. Singh J. A multifaceted topology of patient satisfaction with a hospital. Journal of Health Care Marketing 10:8–21; 1990.
10. Ware JE, Davies AR. Behavioral consequences of consumer dissatisfaction with medical care. Evaluation and Program Planning. 6:301–7; 1083.
11. Meterko, M. Overview: the evolution of customer feedback in health care. Journal of Quality Improvement. 22:5:307–310, 1999.
12. National Center for Health Statistics. Health U.S. Hyattsville, MD: U.S. Department of Health and Human Services, Centers for Disease Control and Prevention 1999.
13. Vickery DM, Glaszewski TJ, Wright EC, Kalmer H. The effect of self-care interventions on the use of medical service within a Medicare population. Medical Care. 26:580–588, 1988.
14. National Committee for Quality Assurance, accessed July 2000 http://www.NCQA.org, 1999.
15. US Government Accounting Office. Consumer Health Informatics: Emerging Issues. Washington, DC: US Government Accounting Office; 1996. Publication GAO/AIMD-96-86.
16. Harris poll #76, December 22, 1999. Online population growth surges to 56% of all adults. http://www.harrisinteractive.com/harris_poll/index.asp?PID=9 accessed June 2000.
17. FIND/SVP Inc. The 1997 American Internet User Survey. New York, NY: Cyber Dialogue, Inc. 1997.
18. CyberDialogue. Impacts of the internet on the doctor-patient relationship; the rise of the internet health consumer. http://www.cyberdialogue.com/pdfs/wp/wp-cch-1999-doctors.pdf, Accessed August 2000, 1999.
19. National Library of Medicine Publication, Gratefully Yours. 1998; Mar/Apr:5. Bethesda, MD.
20. National Managed Health Care Congress (NMHCC). Results of latest managed-care IT study from Microsoft, NMHCC, Dorenfest and Compaq shows internet is key to addressing IT challenges. http://www.microsoft.com/industry/health/news/nmhccPR.asp accessed June 2000.

21. Staggers N, Thompson CR, Happ B, Thomas CR. An operational model for patient-centered informatics. Computers in Nursing 1999 Nov–Dec; 17(6): 278–85.

22. Nahm, R, Poston, I. Measurement of the effects of an integrated point-of-care computer system on quality of nursing documentation and patient satisfaction. Computers in Nursing 18, 5, 220–229, 2000.

23. Holzmer WI, Henry SG. Computer supported vs manually generated nursing care plans; a comparison of patient problems, nursing interventions, and AIDS patient outcomes. Computers in Nursing, 10: 199–24, 1992.

24. Hendrickson G, Kouner CT, Kinckman JR, Finkler SA. Implementation of a variety of computerized bedside nursing information systems in 17 New Jersey Hospitals. Computers in Nursing, 13: 96–102, 1995.

25. Doak CC, Doak LG, Root JH. Teaching patients with low literacy skills. 2nd ed. Philadelphia, JB Lippincott-Raven Publishers, 1996.

26. Kreuter MW, Farrell D, Olevitch L, Brennan L. Tailoring Health Messages: Customizing Communication with Computer Technology. Earlbaum Publishers, N.J. 2000.

27. Wise PH, Pietroni RG, Bhatt VB, Bond CS, Hirst S, Hooker RJ. Development and evaluation of a novel patient information system. J R Soc Med 89: 557–560, 1996.

28. Glascoe FP, Oberklaid F, Dworkin PH, Trimm F. Brief approaches to educating patients and parents in primary care. Pediatrics 101:1068, 1998.

29. Anderson JE, Morrell DC, Avery AJ, Watkins CJ. Evaluation of a patient education manual. British Medical Journal 281:924–925, 1980.

30. Casey R, McMahon F, McCormick MC. Fever therapy: educational intervention for parents. Pediatrics 73:600–603, 1984.

31. Roberts CR, Imrey PB, Turner JD. Reducing physician visits for colds through consumer education. JAMA 250:1986–1989, 1993.

32. Bhopal RS, Gilmour WH, Fallon CW, Bhopal JS, Hamilton I. Evaluation of a practice information leaflet. Family Practice 7:132–137, 1990.

32. Chamorro, T, and Apelbaum, J. Informed consent: nursing issues and ethical dilemmas. Oncology Nursing Forum 15(6):803–8, 1998.

33. Feste C, Anderson RM. Empowerment: from philosophy to practice. Patient Education Counseling 26:139–144, 1995.

33. McVea K, Venugopal M, Crabtree B: The organization and distribution of patient education materials in family medicine practices. Journal of Family Practice 49(4), 319–326, 2000.

34. Bandura, A. Social foundations of thought and action: A social cognitive theory. Englewood Cliffs, NJ, Prentice-Hall, 1986.

35. Prochaska, JO, DiClemente CC, Norcross JC. In search of how people change, applications to addictive behaviors. American Psychology 47:1102–1114, 1992.

36. Science Panel on Interactive Communication and Health. Wired for Health and Well-Being: the Emergence of Interactive Health Communication. Washington, DC: US Department of Health and Human Services, US Government Printing Office, April 1999.

38. Nielsen, E., and Sheppard, M.S. Television as a patient education tool: a review of its effectiveness. Patient Education and Counseling 11(1):3–16, Feb 1988.
39. Alkhateeb W, Lukeroth CJ, Riggs M. A comparison of three educational techniques used in a venereal disease clinic. Public Health Rep. 1975 Mar–Apr; 90(2):159–64.
40. Rosenthal, AR, Zimmerman, JF, and Tanner, J. Educating the glaucoma patient. British Journal of Ophthalmology 67:814–17, 1983.
41. Marshall WR, Rothenberger LA, Bunnell SL. The efficacy of personalized audiovisual patient-education materials. Journal of Family Practice 1984 Nov;19(5):659–63.
42. Mazzuca SA, Moorman NH, Wheeler ML, Norton JA, Fineberg NS, Vinicor F, Cohen SJ, Clark CM Jr. The diabetes education study: a controlled trial of the effects of diabetes patient education. Diabetes Care. 1986 Jan–Feb; 9(1):1–10.
43. Lewis, Deborah. Computer-based approaches to patient education: a review of the literature. Journal of the American Medical Informatics Association 5:4:272–282, 1999.
44. AHCPR (Agency for Health Care Policy and Research). Consumer health informatics and patient decision-making. Final report. Rockville, MD: US Department of Health and Human Services, Agency for Health Care and Policy Research AHCPR publication 98-N001, 1997.
45. Griest JH, Kelin MH, Van Cura LJ. A computer interview for psychiatric patient target symptoms. Archives of General Psychiatry 29:247–253, 1973.
46. Millstein SSG, Irwin CE Jr. Acceptability of computer-acquired sexual histories in adolescent girls. Journal of Pediatrics 103(5) 815–819, 1983.
47. Paperny DM. Computerized health assessment and education for adolescent HIV and STD prevention in health care settings and schools. Health Education and Behavior 24(1) 54–70, 1997.
48. Erdman, HP, Klein MH, Greist JH. Direct patient computer interviewing. Journal of Consulting Clinical Psychology. 53:760–773, 1985.
49. Kieschnick T, Adler, L, Jimison H. 1996 Health Informatics Directory, Williams & Wilkins, 1996.
50. Cornelius L, Beauregard K, Cohen J. Usual sources of medical care and their characteristics. Agency for Health Care Policy and Research Pub. 91–0042, Rockville, MD: Public Health Service 1991.
51. Ferguson T. Health online. How to find health information, support groups, and self-help communities in cyberspace. Reading, MA: Addison-Wesley Publishing Company; 1996.
52. Klemm P, Reppert K, Visich L. A nontraditional cancer support group: the Internet. Computers in Nursing 16: 31–36, 1998.
53. King S. Analysis of electronic support groups for recovering addicts (online). Available at: http://www.concentric.net/-astorm/elect.html. Accessed: July, 2000.
54. Fernsler JI, Manchester LJ. Evaluation of a computer based cancer support network. Cancer Practice 5:46–51, 1997.

55. Winzelberg A. The analysis of an electronic support group for individuals with eating disorders. Computers in Human Behavior 13:393–407, 1997.
56. Finn J. An exploration of helping processes in an online self-help group focusing on issues of disability. Health and Social Work. 24:220–231, 1999.
57. White MH, Dorman SM. Online support for caregivers; analysis of an internet Alzheimer mailgroup. Computer in Nursing 18:4:168–176, 2000.
58. Alemi F, Mosavel M, Stephens RC, Ghadiri A, Krishnaswamy J, Thakkar H. Electronic self-help and support groups. Medical Care 10(suppl):0S32–OS44, 1996.
59. Gustafson DH, Bosworth K, Hawkins RP, Boberg EW, Bricker E. CHESS: a computer-based system for providing information, referrals, decision support and social support to people facing medical and other health-related crises. Proceedings of Annual Symposium on Computer Applications in Medical Care. 1992:161–165.
60. Weinberg N, Schmale JD, Uken J, Wessel K. Computer-medicated support groups. Social Work with Groups. 17:43–54, 1995.
61. Feenberg AL, Licht JM, Kane KP, Moran K, Smith RA. The online patient meeting. Journal of Neurological Science 139(suppl):129–131, 1996.
62. Culver JD, Gerr F, Frumkin H. Medical information on the Internet: a study of an electronic bulletin board. Journal of General Internal Medicine. 12:466–470, 1997.
62. McClung HJ, Murray RD, Heitlinger LA. The internet as a source for current patient information. Pediatrics 101:E2, 1998.
63. Impicciatore P, Pandolfini C, Casella N, Bonati M. Reliability of health information for the public on the world wide web; systematic survey of advice on managing fever in children at home. British Medical Journal. 314:1875–1879, 1997.
64. Eysenbach G, Diepgen, TL. Towards quality management of medical information on the internet: evaluation, labelling, and filtering of information. BMJ. 1998 Nov 28;317(7171):1496–500.
65. Coiera E. Information epidemics, economics and immunity on the internet. British Medical Journal 317:1469–1470, 1998.
66. Greenfield S, Kaplan S, Ware J. Expanding patient involvement in care: effects on patient outcomes. Annuals of Internal Medicine 102:520–528, 1985.
67. Brody DS, Miller SM, Lerman CE, Smith DG, Caputo GC. Patient perception of involvement in medical care: relationship to illness attitudes and outcomes. Journal of General Internal Medicine 4:506–511, 1989.
68. Ambre J, Guard R, Perveiler FM, Renner J, Ripen H. White paper: criteria for assessing the quality of health information on the internet. http://hitiweb .mitretek.org/docs/criteria.html, accessed June 2000, 1999.
69. Kim P, Eng TR, Deering MJ, Maxfield A. Published criteria for evaluating health related web sites: review. BMJ. 1999 Mar 6;318(7184):647–9.
70. McNab A, Anagnostelis B, Cooke A. Never mind the quality, check the badgewidth! Ariadne 9: http://www.xo.com/, 1997.

71. Jadad AR, Gagliardi A. Rating health information on the internet. JAMA 279: 611–614, 1998.
72. *Consumer Reports,* Finding medical help online. 27–31, 1997.
73. Kaplan SH, Greenfield S, Ware JE. Assessing the effects of physician-patient interactions on the outcomes of chronic disease. Medical Care 27:3:110–127, 1989.
74. Juge CF, Assal JP. Designing computer-assisted instruction programs for diabetic patients; how can we make them really useful? Proceedings of Annual Symposium on Computer Applications in Medical Care; 215–219, 1992.
75. Marrero DG, Kronz KK, Golden MP, Wright JC, Orr DP, Fineberg NS. Clinical evaluation of computer assisted self monitoring of blood glucose system. Diabetes Care 12: 345–350, 1989.
77. Nishimoto M, Kobayashi Y, Kuribayashi S, Takabayashi K, Yoshida S, Satomoro, Y. Computer-assisted instruction for diabetic patients using multimedia environment on a Macintosh computer. In: Grobe SJ, Pluyter-Wenting ESP (eds). Nursing Informatics: An international overview in a technological era. Amsterdam, The Netherlands: Elsevier 423, 1994.
78. Keoun B. At last, doctors begin to jump online. Journal of National Cancer Institute. 88:1610–1612, 1996a.
79. Bero L, Jadad AR. How consumers and policy makers can use systematic reviews for decisionmaking. Annals of Internal Medicine. 127:37–42, 1997.
80. Borowitz SM, Wyatt JC. The origin, content and workloads of e-mail consultations. JAMA 280:1321–1324, 1998.
81. Hebert H. The impact of computer-based information systems on quality patient care. Clinical Performance and Quality Health Care, 3:3:169–173, 1995.
82. Drazen EL. Methods of evaluating costs of automated hospital information systems. In: Blum BI ed., Information systems for patient care. New York: Springer-Verlag 1019, 1984.
83. Wang CC. The future of health promotion: talkin' technology blues. Health Promotion Practice. 1:1:77–88, 2000.
84. Eng TR, Maxfield A, Patrick K, Deering MJ, Ratzan SC and Gustafson DH. Access to health information and support: a public highway or a private road? JAMA, 280:15:1371–1375, 1998.
85. NHF (National Health Foundation). Consumer health information preference survey of California Internet users. Los Angeles, CA: National Health Foundation; 1998. Available at: http://www.nationalhealthfdt.org/What_s_New /Survey/survey.html. Accessed July 2000.
86. Brownson, K. Patient handouts? We're wasting our time. RN 56:7:88 1993.
87. US Department of Education. Adult Literacy in America: National Adult Literacy Survey, document #065–000–00588–3, 1993.
88. Jastak Associates Inc., Wide Range Achievement Test (WRAT3), http://www .widerange.com/aboutus.html, 1993.
89. Davis TC, Crouch MA, Long SW, Jackson RH, Bates P, George RB, Bairnsfather LE. Rapid estimate of adult literacy in medicine: a shortened screening instrument. Family Medicine 25(6):391–395, 1993.

90. Buhle EI, Goldwein JW, Benjamin I. Oncolink: a multimedia oncology information resource on the internet. Proceeds of Annual Symposium on Computers in Applied Medical Care. 103–107, 1994.
91. Wingerson L, Simon K, Northrup L, Restino A, eds. Patient Resources on the Internet: 1997 Guide for Health Care Professionals. New York, NY: Faulkner & Gray, Inc.; 1997.
92. OTA (Office of Technology Assessment). Bringing health care online: the role of information technologies. Washington, DC: US Government Printing Office; Report OTA-ITC-624, 1995.
93. Barry MJ, Fowler FJ, Mulley AG, Henderson JV, Wennberg JE. Patient reactions to a program designed to facilitate patient participation in treatment decisions for benign prostatic hyperplasia. Medical Care. 33:771–782, 1995.
94. Firshein J. US Physicians' malpractice data goes on Internet. Lancet 349:1155, 1997.
95. Gustafson DH, Hawkins R, Boberg E, Pingree S, Serlin RE, Graziano F, Chan CL. Impact of a patient-centered, computer-based health information /support system. American Journal of Preventive Medicine. 1999 Jan: 16(1):1–9.
96. Meyer H. Information systems: surfing the net for a health plan. Hospital Health Network 70:37–38, 1996.
97. Wennberg J. Shared decision making and multimedia. In: Harris LM, ed. Health and the new media: technologies transforming personal and public health. Mahwah, NJ: Lawrence Erlbaum Associates, Publishers, 109–126, 1995.
98. Campbell MK, DeVellis BM, Strecher VJ, Ammerman AS, DeVellis RF, Sandler RS. Improving dietary behavior; the effectiveness of tailored messages in primary care settings. American Journal of Public Health. 84:783–787, 1994.
99. Krishna S, Balas EA, Spencer DC, Griffin JZ, Boren SA. Clinical trials of interactive computerized patient education; implications for family practice. Journal of Family Practice. 45:23–33, 1997.
100. Robinson TN. Community health behavior change through computer network health promotion; preliminary findings from Stanford Health-Net. Comput Methods Programs Biomed. 30:137–144, 1989.
101. Skinner CS, Siegfried JC, Kegler MC, Strecher VJ. The potential of computers in patient education. Patient Education Counseling. 22:27–34, 1993.
102. Strecher VJ, Kreuter M, Den Boer DJ, Kobrin S, Hospers HJ, Skinner CS. The effects of computer-tailored smoking cessation messages in family practice settings. The Journal of Family Practice 1994 Sep: 39(3) 290–291.
103. Bluming A, Mittelman PS. Los Angeles free-net: an experiment in interactive telecommunication between lay members of the Los Angeles community and health care experts. Bulletin of Medical Library Association. 84: 217–222, 1996.
104. Gleason NA. A new approach to disordered eating—using an electronic bulletin board to confront social pressure on body image. Journal of American College Health 44:78–80, 1995.

105. Weinberg N, Schmale J, Uken J, Wessel K. Online help: cancer patients participate in a computer-medicated support group. Health and Social Work. 21:24–29, 1996.
106. Peters R, Sikoski R. Digital dialogue. Sharing information and interest on the internet. JAMA 277:1258–1260, 1997.
107. Scolamiero SJ. Support groups in cyberspace. MD Computing 14:12–17, 1997.
108. White BJ, and Madara EJ, eds. The self-help sourcebook: your guide to community and online support groups. 6th edition. Denville, NJ; American Self-Help Clearinghouse; 1998.
109. Ferguson T. Health care in cyberspace: patients lead a revolution. The Futurist. 31:29–33, 1997.
110. Shah NB, Der E, Ruggerio C, Heidenreich PA, Massie BM. Prevention of hospitalizations for heart failure with an interactive home monitoring program. American Heart Journal 135:373–378, 1998.
111. Balas EA, Austin SM, Mitchell JA, Ewigman BG, Bopp KD, Brown GD. The clinical value of computerized information services. A review of 98 randomized clinical trials. Archives of Family Medicine. 5:271–278, 1996.
112. Fries JF, Koop CE, Sokolov J, Beadle CE, Wright D. Beyond health promotion: Reducing need and demand for medical care. Health Affairs 17:70–84, 1998.
113. Kane B, Zands DZ. Guidelines for the clinical use of electronic mail with patients. Journal of the American Medical Informatics Association. 5:104–111, 1998.
114. Mullich J. Patient heal thyself. Healthcare Informatics 27–32, 1997.

10
Workflow Automation with Electronic Medical Records

CEDRIC J. PRIEBE III, M.D., AND ERIC ROSE, M.D.

Scenario 1

Workflow in the paper-based environment. A patient calls his physician's office to request a refill of hydrochlorothiazide for hypertension. The office receptionist cannot transfer the call to the office nurse, because she is on hold with a managed care company. The receptionist writes down the patient's name and "hyacordide," his best guess at the medication name, but it is 45 minutes until he can give the message to the office nurse because he is tied up at the front desk checking in patients. When the nurse gets the message, she needs to call the patient back because what the receptionist wrote down doesn't seem to correspond to any medication she knows. She gets the correct information from the patient and consults her office refill protocol. This tells her that the medication requested requires periodic monitoring of serum potassium and blood pressure levels, so she leaves her station to look for the patient's chart. After a 30-minute search, she finds the chart in the office lunchroom and sees that the patient had a normal potassium level and blood pressure two weeks previously. Per her refill protocol, she calls in a 3-month refill of the medication to the patient's pharmacy. She fills out a paper "refill slip" developed for this purpose by the office. She tapes it onto a page of the patient's chart. Finally, she puts the chart in the physician's in-box for the slip to be cosigned. However, the slip falls out, and no record of the refill remains in the patient's chart. The physician takes the chart, along with the others in her box, and accidentally leaves them in the office lunchroom.

Workflow in the electronic medical record (EMR) environment. A patient calls his physician's office to request a refill of hydrochlorothiazide for hypertension. The office receptionist opens the patient's record in the EMR application and brings up the list of his current medications. He easily identifies hydrochlorothiazide as the medication the patient is requesting and clicks a button on his screen to indicate that a refill is being requested and to electronically transfer the task to the office nurse's EMR "in-box." The office nurse, on hold with a managed care company, checks her inbox and sees the refill request as a new item. She consults her office refill protocol. This tells her that the medication requested requires periodic monitoring of serum potassium and blood pressure, so she clicks on the "laboratory" and "vital signs" sections of the patient's record in the EMR and finds that the patient had a normal potassium level and blood pressure two weeks previously. Per her refill protocol, she calls in a 3-month refill of the medication to the patient's pharmacy, documents her order in the EMR patient record, and clicks on a button to electronically transfer the task to the physician for cosigning. The physician, checking her EMR in-box, sees that the medication was refilled according to the office protocol and cosigns the prescription with a click of the mouse.

Scenario 2

Workflow in the paper-based environment. A physician receives the results (on paper) of a prothrombin time test on one of her patients. The chart, containing a copy of the clinic's anticoagulation care plan, cannot be located. The prothrombin INR value is 2.8. The physician is quite sure the patient is on warfarin, and since the INR value would be in the "therapeutic range" for all indications, initials the lab report and gives it to his nurse to be filed in the patient's chart when it is found.

Workflow in the EMR environment. A physician receives the results in her EMR task list of a prothrombin time test on one of her patients. The prothrombin INR value is 2.8. When she views the results, the EMR also displays the anticoagulation care plan, which shows her that the indication for anticoagulation is a deep vein thrombosis that occurred over 5 months ago, and the patient is to discontinue warfarin 3 weeks later. The EMR also displays an automated alert that the current INR value, though within the therapeutic range, has sharply increased from the previous value of 2.1. With a click of her mouse, she invokes the system's drug-drug interaction engine, which shows her that a recent prescription for erythromycin might be increasing the effect of warfarin. She changes the "Frequency of prothrombin time checks" setting on the care plan display from "every 8 weeks" to "every 1 week" and sends an electronic message to her nurse to arrange the weekly prothrombin time checks and make sure the patient knows to stop the warfarin in 3 weeks. The nurse, using a standardized letter template, sends the notice by mail to the patient, and the text of the letter is automatically saved as part of the patient record.

Scenario 3

Workflow in the paper-based environment. A 58-year-old man presents with vague abdominal pain and occasional rectal bleeding. Examination reveals a hard mass in the lower left quadrant of the abdomen and guaiac-positive stool. Colonoscopic biopsy reveals adenocarcinoma, and further workup identifies extensive hepatic metastases. The patient undergoes chemotherapy but dies 3 months later. Review of his chart shows that he had been seen 18 times since age 50, all acute "work-in" visits, and had never been offered colorectal cancer screening.

Workflow in the EMR environment. A 56-year-old man presents for a "same-day add-on" appointment with the clinic's physician assistant for a wrist sprain. The practice's newly installed EMR software alerts the physician assistant that the patient has not had colorectal cancer screening. He hands the patient a fecal occult blood testing kit at the conclusion of the visit. The results are positive, and the physician assistant refers him to a local gastroenterologist for a colonoscopy, which identifies an adenomatous polyp that is excised without complication.

Epilogue. One year later, the EMR software sends an automated alert to the patient's primary physician's EMR task list alerting her that the patient is due once more for fecal occult blood testing. Since the patient's colonoscopy was performed outside the practice, the data were not captured by the EMR's proactive health supervision function. With a click of the mouse, she sends the patient a standardized letter asking him to return for repeat fecal occult blood testing. He calls back rather upset, stating, "That gastroenterologist told me I didn't need to do those cards anymore, just get another colonoscopy in 5 years. Why don't you people talk to each other?"

Introduction

Workflow Definitions

The concept of "workflow" originated in the business literature in the early 1970s in the context of large organizations where projects would be passed from one individual or team to another, each performing a specified task or set of tasks toward completion of the project. This "flow" of work tended to be inflexible and often unidirectional, and there were often institutional and geographic barriers to close collaboration between those working at different stages in the flow. In subsequent decades, rapid advances in information technology allowed easier and faster collaboration and communication among groups working together. With this trend, the concepts of "workflow management" and "workflow automation" received correspondingly greater attention. Businesses began to design workflows with greater detail and flexibility and to implement them using computer software designed especially for that purpose. In addition, areas outside the traditional business environment, including clinical medicine, began to take the same approach.

For the purposes of this chapter, we will define "workflow" as a pattern of performing a multistep task in roughly the same way over multiple instances. "Workflow automation," then, is the use of software to facilitate workflows by presenting the right information at the right time to individuals or groups and recording the presentation and the actions taken by the recipient(s). It is important to point out that although workflows are often thought of as products of a structured design process, many workflows develop spontaneously through the initiative of those performing the tasks involved. In practice, most workflows are the combined product of a priori design and modification by those who carry them out. Modification of workflows by task performers can result either from valid insights that failed to occur to the designer ("adaptive" modification) or from misunder-

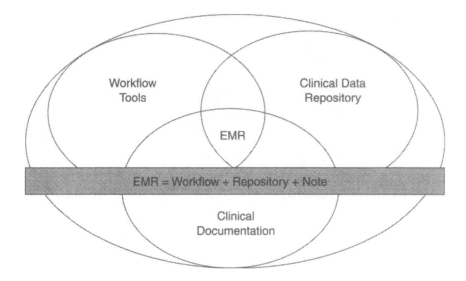

FIGURE 10.1. Workflow tools as a component of an EMR system.

standing of the intended workflow or other aspects of the task at hand ("maladaptive" modification).

   Workflow automation is usually a key component of EMR software, which integrates such functions with patient data repository and tools to document care (Figure 10.1) In this chapter, we describe the variety of workflow tools currently incorporated into many EMR systems and the impact they may have on clinical workflows. We also describe challenges to automating clinical workflows and suggest strategies for success in doing so. All the workflow tools discussed are incorporated into currently available software. However, not all tools are included in all EMR systems. Given the absence of detailed published reports and rigorously controlled studies, statements on the impact of workflow automation are based on the experience of the authors.

Goals of Automating Office-Based Workflow

The success of workflow automation depends on its ability to both facilitate conventional tasks and transform the work itself toward improved and previously impossible outcomes. The goal is not simply to "pave the cowpaths" of existing manual processes by rote automation. There is both the opportunity and the need to reevaluate current clinical and administrative processes in the selection and implementation of an EMR system. Among the purported benefits of workflow automation in clinical settings are the following:

• *Greater clarity of intended workflows and consistency of workflow execution*
  If properly designed, automated workflows have the potential to reduce confusion and maladaptive modification of workflows.

- *Improved efficiency*   By increasing accessibility and ease of transmission of information, workflow automation may speed completion of clinical tasks, resulting in lower costs, greater patient satisfaction, and potentially improved clinical outcomes.
- *Improved task management*   Workflow automation software often includes features that allow sorting of tasks by quantifiable characteristics (e.g. date) or reminders to a user if a task remains unfinished for too long.
- *Better documentation of clinical tasks*   Software that generates documentation as a by-product of a clinical workflow may help support quality care and appropriate compensation for clinical services and may reduce malpractice risks.
- *Automated decision support*   Software that can "sense" clinical aspects of a particular situation can provide appropriate medical knowledge to improve the quality of care.
- *Population-based monitoring*   Capture of workflow events as discrete elements can facilitate aggregate reporting and surveillance within a population for the purposes of health and disease management.
- *Monitoring of task performance*   Software that can track events across a workflow can be used to reliably monitor productivity or to reassign work among members of a workgroup.
- *Rapid implementation of system-wide changes*   When necessary, automated workflows may be modified instantaneously across an institution, reducing errors and delays in adopting the revised workflows.

Features of EMR Workflow Systems

General Characteristics

- *Generic tools applied across all workflows*   If a single tool or feature is useful across multiple workflows, reuse of it as a generic tool is better than forcing users to learn multiple variations of common actions. Several such generic workflow tools are described in this section.
- *Group- and user-level configuration*   Workflow systems need to be highly configurable to match local variations. These configurations need to be applicable to both individual users and aggregates of users. Certain group-level configurations need to accommodate user role–specific behavior, such as the need to configure types of actions a nurse practitioner can perform on a medication renewal task. Other group-level configurations need to accommodate organizational differences based on specialty or business need, such as the different ways a pediatric office and an orthopedic office handle telephone calls from patients.
- *Urgency-based behavior*   The behavior of functionality within a workflow system needs to be modulated by the urgency of the work it represents. For example, a task representing a critical serum potassium value needs to behave differently from a task representing a telephone call from a pharmaceutical detail representative.

- *Documentation as by-product of workflow*   Whenever possible, formal documentation, if required, should be a by-product of the execution of the workflow, not a separate activity. For instance, the actions required to select and review a patient's laboratory result should be sufficient to document its verification in the medical record.
- *Typical and exceptional cases*   All workflows supported by EMR systems should accommodate both the most frequent patterns of use as well as the rare cases or exceptions. The former needs to be tuned for efficiency and the latter for flexibility.

Time Management Tools

Helping clinicians know what needs to be done and when to do it is a central feature of EMR workflow tools. In the ambulatory setting, this commonly means giving the clinician a view of the schedule of patient appointments. While the creation of patient appointments and the necessary collection of demographic and insurance information is usually managed by nonclinical users within separate software systems called practice management systems, the workflow tools within an EMR system need to receive that information and render it in views appropriate for the clinician. Two such views are the schedule of patient appointments with a specific provider and patient appointments for a collection of providers in a location. The scale of time displayed should be adjustable, ranging from a half-day or session view to a day, week, and month view. The attributes of the patient appointment displayed may vary with the view selected and depends on the degree of integration with the practice management system. Generally useful attributes include patient name, age, sex, reason for visit and appointment status (e.g., pending, arrived, cancelled, rescheduled). A view of all patient appointments scheduled for a specific location on the current day can provide a useful display of patient flow in that location analogous to the departure and arrival displays at an airline terminal. Visual indicators in the clinicians' view of their schedule, such as colors or icons used to indicate the status of the appointment and other workflow features specific to the patient, including the presence and number of pending tasks or orders, are helpful prompts to action.

The schedule view is frequently the means by which a user selects a patient for further actions within the system. For example, seeing that a patient has an appointment later in the day, the provider may want to review recent results for that patient. To support this, the system should allow selection of the active patient from the provider's view of the schedule and easy transition to other EMR functions with the selected patient.

Finally, as more and more physicians manage their personal schedules and calendars using personal information management (PIM) features of personal digital assistant (PDA) devices and group scheduling systems, the ability to combine and overlay patient and nonpatient appointments and activities into common views is increasingly valuable.

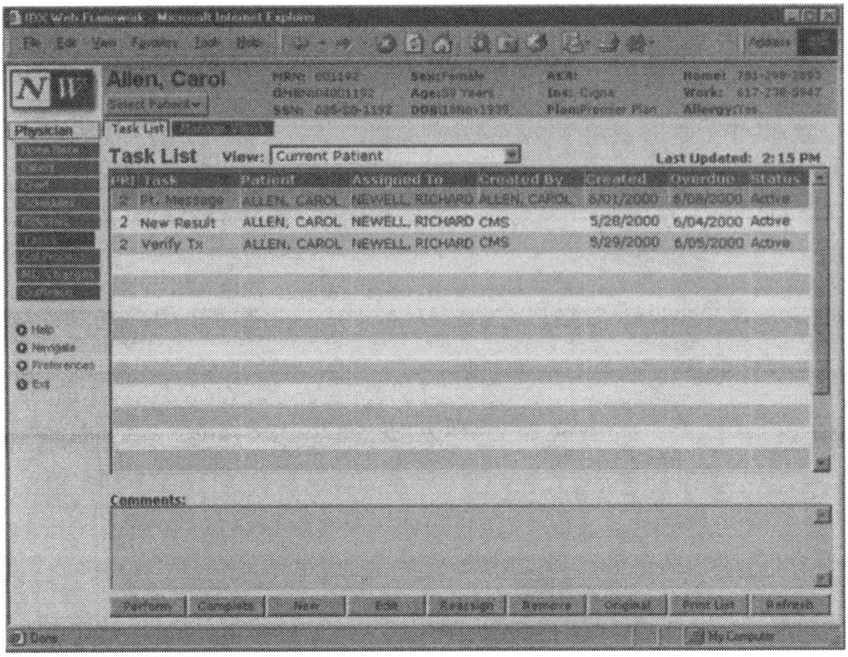

FIGURE 10.2. Example of task list management for tasks specific to a fictitious patient. Used with permission from ChannelHealth® from their ResultWorks™ product.

Task Management Tools

Inherent in every EMR workflow system is a design and data structure that represents a unit of work. For the purposes of this discussion, these atoms of work are described as tasks and the tools that help the user manage them as task management tools. Categories of tasks relevant to an EMR system include follow-up calls to patients, medication renewal requests, transcription verification, and diagnostic test result review. Instances of tasks within each category may carry additional attributes, such as identification of the relevant patient and the assigned provider, the creation date and time, the priority, the status, and so on. As the "working" of tasks is usually done in batches, a task list is the fundamental workspace for task management.

Tasks are often assigned to a specific individual user. However, multiple users may be required to process a given task throughout its life cycle, or the assigned user may be unavailable to perform it. Thus, the task management system becomes a conduit through which work is routed and shared between clinical and administrative users within a practice group. In fact, it is helpful to visualize all the tasks for all the patients receiving care from a group of providers as contained within a common virtual "sea of tasks." From this sea, each user or team of users selects which tasks they want to include on their current task list by the application of filters and sorts (Figure 10.2). Optimally, these task filters and sorts are both preconfigured and defined by the user at the time of viewing. Such a system of task management can enable the sharing of task performance among users on a team or between users in a cross-coverage setting.

Several features can greatly facilitate the performance of tasks in the clinical office setting. First, if the work necessary to complete the task is performed by functionality within the EMR system, then a single user action on that task should navigate the user to the appropriate forms and the appropriate context applied to facilitate the performance of the work. Beyond that, if the system is able to sense the completion of the work represented by the task, then the task status and task list should update automatically. The category of task should determine other behaviors of the task as well. For example, patient callback tasks may be required to trigger overdue alert tasks to the originating user if the task is not completed within a specified time, while a transcription verification task may not. Finally, easy citation of some or all of the information contained within a task instance into a clinical note enables the timely and completed documentation of care in the patient's medical record.

Event Notification

The workflow tools of EMR systems can facilitate care delivery in the primary care office only if the relevant personnel are notified promptly of tasks and events that need attention. Multiple communication and alerting methods are available for this within both the EMR application user interface and external modalities such as pagers, facsimile, telephony, and voice and electronic mail systems. Optimally, the routing of an event notification is determined by rules specific to the event type and the user's time-sensitive preferences. For instance, the desired routing of a laboratory test result may be to create a "review result" task assigned to the ordering physician. However, if the result is abnormal, that task assumes an "urgent" status, which includes it in the task list of the office's triage nurse. If the result is in the panic range, a telephone call is made to the office and the ordering provider receives an alphanumeric page message alerting her to the event. Often, for reasons of security and confidentiality, external methods of event notification such as pager, fax, and e-mail should simply alert the user that important information needs their attention and thus drives them to a reliably authenticated EMR session. Within the EMR system, the presence and quantity of workflow items, particularly tasks of different types, can be effectively represented using graphical meters and iconic indicators similar to those on the dashboard of an automobile. Such dashboard indicators of workflow tool status can be presented both at the start of every log-in session or as a persistent frame in the user interface.

Messaging

Messaging between and among clinical and administrative resources in the primary care office is a critical workflow process. The ability for one user to inform

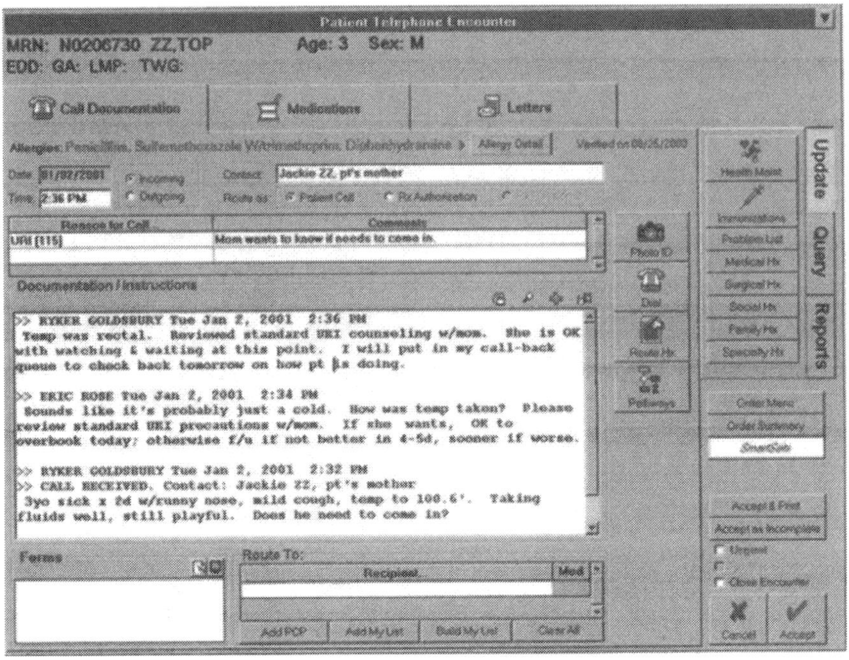

FIGURE 10.3. View of a "telephone encounter" screen in an EMR system, showing an exchange between a physician and triage nurse regarding an ill patient who has contacted the clinic by telephone. Used with permission from Epic Systems Corporation.

another user of work done or the need for work to be done for a patient without interrupting the second user enables the "batch" processing of work by both sender and receiver. Without such means of asynchronous communication between clinicians, the office setting would be chaos. Every primary care office has several messaging processes—the paper mailbox, the paper message box, notes affixed to patient charts stacked with other charts, a voice mail system, one or more electronic mail accounts, and so on. The cost, however, of so many in-boxes is an increase in the average turnaround time for all work, as each in-box can be attended to only so often, and there is a loss of any ability to track the status of work both in particular and in aggregate. In addition, many messaging systems, such as electronic and voice mail, are person-to-person communications. While this serves the purposes of personal messages, much of office-based primary care is conducted in multidisciplinary and/or multiprovider teams where the addressed provider or clinician may not be on duty and attending their inboxes with the frequency necessary to provide adequate turnaround time.

To realize the benefits of asynchronous messaging without the costs of multiple personal in-boxes, many EMR systems utilize task management tools as a formal, secure messaging environment (Figure 10.3). This allows the sender to attach a formal task to a message or reassign a task with a message when appropriate. It also provides the recipient user a single in-box or task list capable of filtering and sorting to display the desired queue of formal tasks and informal messages and with it gain all the benefits of task navigation and documentation previously described.

One newer trend in EMR messaging functionality is to include the patient in this communication network, usually via a World Wide Web–based interface. Using this functionality, patients can be apprised of results, reminded of appointments and can request medication prescription renewals.

Call Processing

Every primary care setting provides some degree of care and/or service to patients via the telephone. In fact, many workflow processes in the office setting are initiated by a telephone call from a patient or about a patient. For efficient use of the telephone, a call-processing feature is a necessary workflow tool in an EMR system. The initial need is to support the call taker in the collection and validation of information from the caller. It can be facilitated by utilizing data already present in the EMR and practice management systems. As call takers are frequently interrupted and calls are frequently passed from one call taker to another, a shared queue of inbound calls is helpful. Depending on the degree of service to be provided via the telephone, additional functionality can be presented to the call taker. For example, demand management tools that assist the call taker in an interview, assessment, and either self-resolution through reassurance or patient education can be made available. A more common approach is the simple recognition of services requested, such as an appointment request, a medication renewal request, or a medical question and an assignment of the work to the appropriate resource.

Patient Lists

The final generic workflow tool with EMR systems to be discussed here is a facility to generate and maintain multiple lists of patients. As a primary care office sets out to automate one or more clinical workflows it is often surprising to discover how many different lists of patients are maintained in a variety of manual ways. Different from task lists, in which each task item represents a unit of work that may or many not pertain to a patient, patient lists are more loosely defined sets of patients compiled for a variety of different reasons. Some patient lists may define ongoing or temporary coverage lists, such as the patients currently admitted to an in-patient facility or on a consultation service. Other patient lists may represent the presence or absence of a data state specific to each patient on the list, such as the set of patients in a practice group that meet the inclusion criteria for a clinical trial or who are in need of yearly influenza vaccine.

Given the ubiquitous need for patient lists in many clinical workflows, a generic set of patient list management tools is desirable in an EMR system. This facility includes the ability to manage a list of lists, some of which are personal lists (seen and maintained only by a specific user), others of which are shared in an organization or across the entire enterprise. Patients can be added to any of these lists either by an *ad hoc* selection or through user-defined queries for specific patient data. Once a patient list is generated or maintained, a user may wish to create in batch a similar task for all patients on the list to trigger completion of subsequent work in the EMR system. Similarly, it is at other times helpful to export a patient list to other office automation software systems such as spreadsheet or word processing applications.

Challenges in Clinical Workflow Automation

Despite the potential benefits of clinical workflow automation in EMR systems, to date such software has had little penetration into primary care delivery settings in the United States. Several clear barriers still exist to broad acceptance—some inherent to the existing software itself, some to other factors.

The productive use of EMR tools requires a significant degree of change to pre-existing office work patterns, both clinical and administrative. In general, users need to form new habits—new ways of obtaining information, new ways of communicating with coworkers, even new ways of moving their bodies in the office. Often the overall success of an EMR implementation depends on the net effect of the initial negative impact on current work patterns plus the positive impact of automated workflow that follows. The transition from paper-based records and workflows to the EMR environment requires substantial effort from clinicians and staff, both in learning to use the software and in creating and adopting new workflows made possible by the software. In addition, the question of how—or whether—a practice incorporates existing paper records into a newly adopted EMR is one for which there is currently no good answer. Many medical practices, with good reason, are hesitant to make such a transition. Even after the transition, in our experience, many users do not fully avail themselves of the workflow tools in EMR systems. Some users, uncomfortable with relying on computerized workflows, may attempt to develop parallel paper-based workflows to avoid data loss or missed communication.

Cost has greatly limited the adoption of EMR systems, particularly in small medical practices. In addition to software costs, the most comprehensive EMR systems usually require substantial investments in computer hardware, communications network maintenance, and professional information technology staff. In our experience, cost considerations often cause medical practices to implement an EMR by placing the necessary hardware in only one or two locations in a medical office, which creates tremendous inconvenience in attempting to use the software while seeing patients. Declining hardware and software costs and improvements in wireless technology may ameliorate this problem.

Limitations of the software itself should not be underestimated as a barrier to EMR adoption. Workflow automation embedded in EMR software may be designed by developers unfamiliar with subtleties of the work itself. If workflows are excessively rigid and cannot be altered by those carrying them out, the process of adaptive modification is suppressed. In some cases, software designers may fail to anticipate a desired type of workflow, requiring the user to develop complicated "workarounds" to achieve a desired result. In other instances, workflow automation in EMR systems may result in task management that's "too good." For instance, software that tracks information not easily trackable in a paper-based environment—e.g., unfinished tasks—despite the obvious benefits, creates new categories of work for clinical personnel. Even in situations where extra work is to the benefit of patient and clinician alike (such as an alert to the clinician that a procedure being ordered is not covered by the patient's insurance plan), it may be perceived as undesirable by the clinician.

The reliance on asynchronous communication common in an EMR environment is worth mention. Most automated workflows rely on asynchronous communication but replace workflows that rely on synchronous communication, introducing new delays in the transmission of tasks from one person to another. For instance, clinicians and staff using EMR systems may tend to communicate with the e-mail-like message function of the EMR so as not to interrupt each other, even though doing so often requires more contacts than does verbal communication.

Difficulties in incorporating external data are another barrier to EMR adoption as a workflow tool. With paper-based medical records, incorporating information received from outside the practice (lab reports, letters from consultants, and so on) simply involves slipping a piece of paper into the patient's chart. In an EMR system, such information can always be incorporated as a scanned image, but the data it contains is, of course, not recognizable by the EMR as such. This limits the usefulness of EMR functionality that leverages stored patient data. For instance, when automated clinical reminders are being generated from the patient database, a "false-positive" alert may be generated, as in the third clinical scenario presented at the beginning of the chapter. One area of data capture of paramount importance is laboratory data. The volume of laboratory data flowing into most medical practices is great, and it would not be feasible for office staff to enter such information by hand into an EMR. However, clinical laboratories use a wide variety of data systems, most of which are not designed to export data to an EMR. In most cases where EMR systems are implemented, interfaces between laboratory information systems and EMR systems must be created, which can be a lengthy and expensive process. If direct interfaces from more than one clinical laboratory are built, data views in the EMR that show laboratory data in tabular or graphic format may display such data together. In situations where different laboratories use different assays with different reference ranges for the same test, an erroneous impression of fluctuation of a lab value may be created.

The development of EMR systems has preceded the development of mature, well-designed data standards for the data they are intended to acquire and manipulate. In some cases, existing data standards are inadequate. For instance, the International Classification of Diseases, Ninth Revision, Clinical Modification (ICD-9-CM) and Current Procedural Terminology (CPT) were not designed for clinical coding in EMR systems and are found by many clinicians to be difficult to use. Nonetheless, they are the currently accepted coding standards for diagnoses and procedures and are required for billing by most third-party payers in the

United States. Because of this, they have become the de facto data standards in EMR systems for recording patients' problem lists, surgical histories, diagnoses for visits, and so on. In other cases, more than one adequate data standard exist but are in conflict. Specifically, efforts have been made to develop diagnostic and procedural data "vocabularies" for use with EMR systems (e.g., SNOMED, MEDCIN). However, there is no current industry standard, and there is little compatibility among those available. Therefore, if an EMR designer incorporates one of these into the EMR, the database may in the future be incompatible with other clinical databases. In some cases, needed data standards are nonexistent. For instance, the absence of data standards for prescription data or health plan formulary data limits the ability of EMR developers to design workflow automation tools for tasks in those areas.

Regulatory barriers to EMR adoption currently exist. One example is that of authentication of electronic orders and documents. EMR workflows enable largely paperless communication between healthcare providers and ancillary services, such as clinical laboratories and radiology departments. For instance, orders may be automatically generated and delivered by facsimile. In the absence of a written signature from the provider, the orders may be challenged as being inauthentic or not meeting regulatory requirements. With the passage in June 2000 of the Electronic Signatures in Global and National Commerce Act, it is likely that this barrier has been lessened. Prescription-writing requirements is another problematic area. There is substantial state-by-state variability in the United States on requirements for medication prescriptions. Some states require special forms to be completed for controlled substances. Some states require that the printed prescription display whether the brand name or generic version of a medication is prescribed. State-specific regulations challenge the EMR system's ability to streamline workflows and make documentation a by-product of task completion.

Conclusion

Automating the clinical workflow of primary care with EMR software holds great promise for improving efficiency and quality of care. Several important barriers still exist, including cost, shortcomings of available software, and skepticism in the medical community itself. Primary care practices planning a transition to EMR use must be prepared for a challenging period of adaptation as they learn to use the software and develop the new habits it requires.

Once the pattern of success derived from office-based workflow tools is experienced and embraced by the users in a primary care practice, unanticipated opportunities for their application are identified. In fact, the best measure of the quality of the task management and other workflow tools in an EMR system may be the degree to which its users modify the system and apply it to uses unanticipated by the designers of the system.

It is possible for primary care practices to automate only a subset of their clinical processes, either by using some but not all functions within an EMR system

TABLE 10.1 Examples of clinical workflows and the impact of cost, time, and quality.

Clinical workflow	Cost impact	Time impact	Quality impact
Prescription management	High	High	High
Test order/result review	High	High	High
Telephone messages	High	High	High
Population management	High	High	High
Service recognition/coding	High	Medium	Low
Referral processing	High	Medium	Low
Patient education	Low	High	Medium
Knowledge source inquiry	Low	Medium	High

or by implementing software that addresses only specific clinical workflows. When selecting which primary care office workflows to automate, we recommend giving priority to those that will benefit most from automation. Table 10.1 lists a subset of these workflows, several of which were addressed in the clinical scenarios. Included is an assessment of the relative consequences of automation on each of these processes of care at a primary care office preparing for an EMR implementation. As is evident, the impact of some workflows on cost, time, and quality are anticipated to be greater than that of others. This analysis should be helpful in the selection of which workflow processes to automate first in a given care setting.

Finally, the description of workflow tools presented here represents only a single point in the evolution of these systems in the healthcare setting. As this evolution proceeds, we envision the broader integration of clinical computing applications, including the workflow tools and EMR systems themselves, into larger networks connecting affiliated institutions and business partners. As the systems of care become more connected, workflow tools will provide the primary care practitioner with a necessary foundation of usability and efficiency. If the result of this progression is a system of community health information networks that span the traditional boundaries of a single patient record at a single institution in a way that promotes individual and community health, workflow tools will have had a large part in their success.

11
Privacy and Security of Patient Information

PAUL D. CLAYTON, PH.D.

Scenario

Imagine your discomfort and eventual lack of patients if the following scenario were to occur. As you and your spouse are in the kitchen doing dishes, you mention that a lovely high school girl consulted you for information on how to discreetly terminate an unplanned pregnancy. One of your children happens to overhear you and the next day remarks to his best friend that it is a tragedy for one of the most popular girls in the school to be pregnant. The friend immediately starts a guessing game of elimination and can tell when your son refuses to confirm or deny the ultimate candidate. Two days later the entire school knows, and ultimately the girl's parents hear the gossip. She knows that you are the only one she told.

This is an example of an inadvertent disclosure that has nothing to do with the computer but illustrates the damage that can be done when privacy is violated. Given the access to on-line records, some people might become nefarious and actively seek data. At our institution, if we did not take precautions, it would be possible for a mother who works as a nurse in one town to see the results of her daughter's boyfriend's chlamydia test even though the boyfriend lives in another town and is seen by a different practitioner.

Before we go further, we should define *privacy*. In the health care arena, privacy is the situation in which an individual desires to limit the disclosure of personal information. *Confidentiality* is the condition in which information is shared or released in a controlled fashion. *Security* is defined as the measures that are taken to protect confidentiality, availability, and integrity of data. In this chapter, we look at the needs for access to patient information and the possibilities for misuse of patient information. Subsequently, we list the actions that can be taken now to ensure that we do not inadvertently cause harm to individuals we seek to serve; finally, we talk about compliance with federal regulations.

There is a long-standing recognition of the need to keep patient records (continuity of care, reminders to the caregiver, legal records, justification for providing certain types of examinations or therapies, and so on). In previous decades, handwritten records were stored in a hospital or the practitioner's office and retrieved when the patient visited. As we began to use the records for additional related information, such as quality assurance and coding for reimbursement, and as single patients be seen to be served by multiple caregivers, often the records could not be found in their expected places. With the advent of the computer, several of the deficiencies of paper records could be potentially overcome. The electronic record is conveniently accessible; even now, it is possible to use the Internet[1,2] or hand-held wireless devices[3] to see information that heretofore could be only in one place at one time. The electronic record is organized. People do not have to look through a 2-inch thick stack of papers to find out if the patient has some condition of which they must be aware (drug allergy, tuberculosis, advance directive, chronic disease, and so on). The computer can provide easy links between problems, drugs, test results, and answers to commonly asked questions about those entities (what is the proper pediatric dose for this drug, and so on). It is possible to use the computer to generate automatic alerts, reminders, and suggestions when standards of care are not being achieved. It is possible to use resulting databases for clinical research[4] and to measure the quality of care and clinical outcomes for various courses of treatment. Automated information systems can also reduce the cost of care[5] and improve the quality of service.

Given these benefits, many providers who see large numbers of patients have invested financial resources with the primary intent of providing convenient access to all or portions of the patient record.[6] Patients have also benefited from these systems because the quality and cost of their care was improved. For instance, the physician is immediately notified of the laboratory test results for elevated enzymes when an acute myocardial infarction is suspected. However, as the extent of medical records has increased and the information passes between organizations, patients have become justifiably concerned that no one see their record who does not have a legitimate reason to do so. They are also asking for accountability so that they can see where their information has gone.

The patient may be harmed by nosy neighbors who gossip, vindictive individuals who are intent on embarrassing or humiliating that person, or by the use of information in a way that can cause economic disadvantage. The latter is of growing concern for the majority of patients. They may be denied a promotion to a high-level executive position if it is known that they have heart disease, or layoffs might unreasonably target those with dependents who have increased health care costs. This concern is increasing as we realize that shortly, our genetic profiles may indicate our individual propensity for future diseases.

Given the simultaneous needs for legitimate access and the desire for confidentiality, the issue becomes one of trade-offs in how many barriers we erect to deter unwarranted access to patient information versus how convenient it is to use: How do we permit convenient access to all necessary data for a person who has a legitimate reason without giving the same privilege to someone else who does not have a valid reason? If we make it very convenient for a busy nurse in the hospital where the patient resides, there may not be enough barriers to prevent access by other people. If we raise the barriers (the patient has a card that a physician must use to gain access permission), then even legitimate stakeholders who are under time pressure in emergency situations will not use the system and the quality of care will deteriorate.

Some general guidelines can be used to solve the trade-off dilemma. Fair information practice is generally founded on several principles: The patient should know that the records are being kept and should have a right to inspect and amend (as appropriate) the content of the records, and the patient should have the right to limit collection and disclosure without consent. As a matter of course, healthcare providers require a patient to consent to the collection and use of information as a condition of receiving treatment, but with the proviso that the use will be limited to legitimate instances of diagnosis and treatment, healthcare operations (quality assessment, scheduling, and so on), reimbursement for services, and research in which no patient-identifiable information will be disclosed to anyone except those who have received permission after providing assurance that they will conduct their research in a way that will not cause patient harm.

The fair information practice principles have recently been codified in regulations issued by the Secretary of Health and Human Services as a consequence of what is known as the HIPAA (Health Insurance Portability and Accountability Act).[7] The development of these regulations was mandated in 1996 because until then, there had been no federal standards or laws that made it a crime to violate medical privacy standards. A pharmacy benefits provider could sell information collected in the course of filling prescriptions without fear of penalty except public outcry. Employers who were paying for their employees' healthcare insurance could find out what they were paying for without penalties for using that information in making personnel decisions unless the affected person hired an attorney and successfully proved damages. The intent of the HIPAA regulations is to clearly indicate what might be considered legitimate use and to prescribe penalties for abuse.

Adapting these broad fair-practice principles and the new regulations to daily situations requires practical measures. We now discuss several well-accepted practices for protecting privacy and ensuring confidentiality. Most of these recommendations are summarized in the work of a committee assembled by the Computer Science and Telecommunications Board of the National Academy of Science. Their report, *For the Record,* was published in 1997.[8]

Authentication. Authentication means that we know who is actually looking at the information. In the era of paper records, someone could put on a white coat and peruse hospital records in many instances without being challenged. The difference in the era of electronic records involves the concept of convenience. One no longer has to physically be present masquerading as a care provider, so curiosity is easier to satisfy. In most cases where the user is accessing data through a terminal connected to the intranet of the enterprise that manages the patient record, a password and a log-on ID suffice to identify a user. There are three main drawbacks to this approach: people can share IDs and passwords; a determined, malevolent hacker could capture the keystrokes; many people do not sign off when they leave a workstation because it is considered the social equivalent of slamming the door in the face of the next waiting user.

Some institutions resort to the concept of "strong" authentication.[9] Strong authentication is used in the banking arena and relies on something you know (the log-on ID and password) *and* something you hold (a physical card or token, a fingerprint, or a retinal scan). This eliminates concurrent sharing, the possibility of stolen passwords, and in some cases the log-off problem (you log off automatically when you remove your token from the computer, as with an automatic teller machine). The disadvantages to this approach are twofold: a physician's home computer, the required special reader device, and the convenience may be impacted if one has to remove a card or token. Several leading institutions mandate the use of log-on ID and password on the locally controlled intranet and strong authentication on the Internet. If a patient can see only his/her own record, the ID and password approach is acceptable. In either case, the data should be encrypted as they are transmitted over the intranet or Internet. Suitable encryption is now rather easily accomplished using the secure socket layer (SSL) protocol.[10]

Access Privileges. Once you know who the user is, it is possible to limit access[11] to information that person might need. The rules that are composed to create access restrictions should depend on five factors: the *relationship* of the user to the patient (primary care provider, nurse who works for the primary care provider, and so on), the location of the terminal being used (nursing floor, emergency room, and so on), the current activity or location of the patient (in the hospital? in the clinic?), the role of the user (radiology technician, pharmacist, and so on), and the type of data to be seen (demographic, psychiatric notes, and so on). These rules must be established as a matter of policy. In most cases, it is assumed that the primary care physician or the nurse who works with the PCP can see any part of any of their patients' data at any time. An institution may also choose to establish a type of data viewable only by the person who entered it.

The individual's role and log-on and password information as well as relationships to other providers are kept in a directory. Directories are increasingly compliant with protocols (lightweight directory access protocol—LDAP) for accessing directory information from the application programs. This means that there is only one location where a user is defined when initially employed or given access privileges and only one place to go when privileges are to be terminated. The individual software applications do not have to have their own copies of that information; they need only access the master user directory for the information they require to evaluate their access rules. This directory approach makes management of the user descriptors much easier.

Many institutions also, by policy, allow a physician or nurse to "break the glass" if they certify that they have a legitimate need to know. This capability allows access for consults, emergencies, cross-coverage, residents who rotate in a fashion that does not allow predetermination, and so on. The institution can also elect by policy to notify the primary care physician via e-mail if the glass is broken when the patient is not currently being treated.

Audit. If you know who is using the system and what they look at, it is possible to construct an audit trail. Using the information in the audit trail and a Web browser, it is possible to let patients see who has accessed their medical record. In addition to the concept of multiple auditors, this capability also sensitizes employees to the fact that their own information-seeking actions are recorded. Obviously, an employee should see only his or her own audit trail because a list of the people (psychiatrists, obstetricians, oncologists, and so on) treating another patient would disclose information that could lead to inferences about that person's health status. Authorized institutional representatives could, on request, provide a patient with a list of individuals who have accessed his or her records. I have been a happy bystander when nurses and residents who had illnesses that they wanted to keep private were overjoyed to see that none of their colleagues had accessed their records. In some instances, it is possible to analyze the audit trail for patterns that indicate that an individual is attracting undue interest, but it is extremely difficult to find in the audit log a single instance of a violation unless someone specifically asks for an accounting. Because the implementation of audit trails is not a feature of many installed systems, the HIPAA regulations do not, at this time, mandate such measures for internal use. However, the regulations do demand an accounting for disclosures other than for healthcare, operations, or reimbursement purposes.

Accountability. In any organization that maintains patient records, it is important to decide who is accountable for setting policy and setting standards. The new HIPAA regulations specifically place this responsibility on the organizational leaders. A chief privacy officer must decide who owns the problem of confidentiality, who will enforce the policies, whom to call when there is a breach, and so on. If the policies are never enforced, the likelihood of a patient being harmed and obtaining a judgment or settlement is increased. In general, these matters are administrative and should not be left by default to technical people who build systems. The HIPAA regulations mandate a clearly identified chief privacy officer. Even in a small clinic or partnership, there must be a clear designation of who is responsible.

Penalties or sanctions should be determined in advance and applied even-handedly via a process that protects employees as well as patients. If a clerk who violates policy is treated differently than a productive surgeon who commits the same type of breach, the organization may be only giving lip service to the principles of confidentiality.

Availability. A system might be vulnerable to outside "denial of service" attacks or insider malicious retaliation; information might be destroyed or made unavailable or made so incomplete that it is unreliable. Denial of service attacks can be mounted by flooding a system with unnecessary messages or by deleting crucial information files. Imagine an instance where an angry relative who was convinced that an organization did not do enough to save someone's life or refused to pay for a possibly miraculous therapy might, as an act of vengeance, hire someone to disable the information system. There are known standards of protection, such as firewalls, redundant pathways, backup procedures, and so on that should be enforced in large organizations. In small offices, internet connections must not permit outsiders access to files. Some might complain that the HIPAA regulations will cause an undue financial burden. But if these simple measures are not applied, it is possible that long-term financial fallout could be even greater. Think what might happen if all accounts receivable information was erased or lost.

Accuracy. A lesser-known issue that may have future implications is the accuracy of the information in records.[12] The electronic format may make it easier for accomplished hackers or employees to delete or change information maliciously or in an attempt to avoid litigation. It should be impossible to repudiate information that is in the patient record. If something has been added or a previous entry was wrong, an addendum should be entered: the previous entries should not be deleted. Some states now have digital signature laws that rely on the encryption of a key, the time of entry, and an abstract of the document in a way that makes it impossible to substitute a forged document at a later time. In the near future, this ability will become commonplace.[13-15]

Awareness. After all is said and done, it is obvious that human integrity is the key to maintaining the confidentiality of patient information. One who discusses confidential information at the dinner table or in the elevator may be unaware of the ethics they are violating. There must be regular and consistent education. At Columbia-Presbyterian Medical Center, the computer is programmed to deliver a message once a year to users of the system on the anniversary of the date they received their access privileges. The message states the policies and asks the user to certify that the policies are understood. At Intermountain Health Care the log-in screen for results review contains the following message: "By logging into this program I certify that I am actively involved in the care of patients whom I access via this program and that I have a legitimate need to see their information. I understand that unjustified access will/may subject me to civil and/or criminal action as well as revocation of my access to this program. IHC will allow the patient and/or the PCP to see that I have accessed the patient's data." Experts consistently say that employees would be justified in claiming ignorance if they are not regularly notified of policies.

This list of action items can act as a checklist. If a small practice feels overwhelmed, it can start slowly. In this business, direction is more important than speed. The *For the Record* [8] committee found that none of the exemplary institutions it was studying had complied with all the recommendations on the list. Most people know they could do more, but until the HIPAA regulations, there has been little pressure to invest scare resources in security issues when the majority of the users are clamoring for more and better means of access. Vendors have indicated that they cannot deliver a turnkey system that incorporates these measures, and they have stated that they cannot charge extra to justify the expense of developing such capabilities. All that is changing. In my opinion, the HIPAA regulations are not onerous or unreasonable at the technical level. For the most part, these regulations require policies and expect the policies to be followed. Even though all the possible technological safeguards may not be in place, a practice can set policy, educate employees, enforce sanctions when breaches occur, and design the information flow in a way that will recognize the future incorporation of these measures. It is also important to remember that there is a point of diminishing returns. Even the best systems can be compromised. However, it is important to do enough to deter the opportunist or nosy neighbor.

Finally it is advisable to critique the current status and to communicate to your employees and patients the standards you have set and to comply with regulations that will become increasingly prevalent. Many computer consultants who are out of work as a result of the largely benign passing of the Y2K milestone are hyping the HIPAA regulations as an urgent indicator for the enlistment of their services. This may be a false trumpet; an institution can assess where they stand and begin to make progress toward ensuring confidentiality without great expenditures for technology. For instance, in recognition of the practical situation that few vendor products that were installed five years ago have audit trails, no such requirement is in evidence in the HIPAA standards. We all recognize that the journey to adequate confidentiality will continue for some time. Those who will most likely be punished are those who have not assessed their situation, put a plan in place, and done the immediately achievable tasks, such as educating employees, setting policy, and appointing a security officer. As patients we will not feel sorry for those who do not start the journey immediately and are penalized as a result.

References

1. Rind DM, Kohane IS, Szolovits P, Safran C, Chueh HC, Barnett GO. Maintaining the confidentiality of medical records shared over the Internet and the World Wide Web. *Ann Intern Med* 1997 Jul 15;127(2):138–41
2. Cimino JJ, Socratous SA, Clayton PD. Internet as clinical information system: Application development using the World Wide Web. *J Am Med Inform Assoc* 1995 Sep–Oct;2(5):273–84.
3. Duncan RG, Shabot MM. Secure remote access to a clinical data repository using a wireless personal digital assistant (PDA). *Proc AMIA Symp* 2000: 210–4.
4. Behlen FM, Johnson SB. Multicenter patient records research: Security policies and tools. *J Am Med Inform Assoc* 1999 Nov–Dec;6(6):435–43
5. Tierney WM, Miller ME, Overhage JM, McDonald CJ. Physician inpatient order writing on microcomputer workstations: Effects on resource utilization. *JAMA* 1993 Jan 20;269(3):379–83.
6. Shortliffe EH. The evolution of electronic medical records. *Acad Med.* 1999 Apr;74(4):414–9.).
7. http://aspe.hhs.gov/admnsimp/final/PvcTxt01.htm
8. *For the Record: Protecting Electronic Health Information.* Washington, DC, National Academy Press, 1997.
9. Masys DR, Baker DB, Barnhart R, Buss T. PCASSO: A secure architecture for access to clinical data via the Internet. *Medinfo* 1998;9 Pt 2:1130–4.
10. http://developer.netscape.com/docs/manuals/security/sslin/contents.htm
11. Bowen JW, Klimczak JC, Ruiz M, Barnes M. Design of access control methods for protecting the confidentiality of patient information in networked systems. *Proc AMIA Annu Fall Symp* 1997:46–50.
12. Burnum JF. The misinformation era: The fall of the medical record. *Ann Intern Med* 1989 Mar 15;110(6):482–4.
13. Smith JP. Authentication of digital medical images with digital signature technology. *Radiology* 1995 Mar;194(3):771–4.

14. Campbell SG, Gibby GL, Collingwood S. The Internet and electronic transmission of medical records. *J Clin Monit* 1997 Sep;13(5):325–34.
15. de Meyer F, Lundgren PA, de Moor G, Fiers T. Determination of user requirements for the secure communication of electronic medical record information. *Int J Med Inf* 1998 Mar;49(1):125–30.)

12
Electronic Billing for the Primary Care Physician

PETER J. HOUSE, M.H.A., AND LYDIA BARTHOLOMEW, M.D.

Scenario

Jimmy comes in for his well-child check. He needs his kindergarten immunizations—tetanus-diptheria (DT), polio, and measles-mumps-rubella (MMR). He also needs a follow-up hemoglobin to see if the iron supplement that he is taking has resolved his anemia. The care Jimmy will get is both routine and complex, and his encounter with his caregivers starts in motion a series of events and creates a cascade of records all in the name of getting the caregivers paid for their services. The office team will do the work to get the practice paid; the provider may never see any of the billing paperwork and may have little understanding of what her office team does. Is that reasonable delegation of a clerical task, or is it a dangerous dereliction of responsibility?

Introduction

Electronic billing (EB) is a mechanism by which providers can bill insurance companies and other third-party payers for care given to patients. There are several ways to participate in EB. In one option, the provider's office fills out a billing form on a computer in the office and submits the claim to the third-party payer via modem. Many of the practice management software packages (e.g., Medical Manager) have an embedded feature that allows EB virtually at the push of a few buttons once the pertinent information is entered. Another option is to send paper claims (or electronic claims) to a clearinghouse that in turn prepares electronic bills and sends them (electronically) to various third-party payers. Some clearinghouses charge fees on a per claim basis, while some insurance companies (Premera in Washington state, for example) provide the service free of charge to their participating physicians. An insurance company providing clearinghouse services will send electronic bills to other insurance companies and third-party payers. A third option is just beginning to be marketed—sending claims to a Web site for processing.

All physicians need to be aware that EB as an important way to save costs and gain more management information for medical practices. More and more, third-party payers are moving to electronic billing, and soon it will be a requirement rather than an option for the physician. A Xerox company spokesman in 2001 estimated that by the end of 2002 it would be possible to replace the entire billing process, including the bills sent to patients, with e-billing. Currently, Medicare accepts only electronic bills from physicians. For physicians in larger practices, where all the administrative details are handled by professional practice managers and office staff, there may be little "need to know" about the details of electronic billing. Nevertheless, it is an integral piece of the financial relationship physicians have with their patients, a relationship that is increasingly complex and strained. In addition, the physician-owner of a practice must have a certain level of understanding of the work that employees are doing. In the final analysis, providers have legal responsibility for the bills that their offices produce, and they are subject to ever-tightening fraud and abuse laws should errors be made in billings.

This chapter explains the basics of EB and gives the practicing physician information about the advantages and disadvantages. We describe the resources and preparation necessary to participate in EB and what to expect in the future.

What Is Electronic Billing?

Electronic billing uses a computer-based system to review, sort, track, and send bills to patients and payers and manage their responses. Elements of an EB system can include the following:

- Determination of patient's eligibility in the health plan
- Electronic claims processing (the central topic of this chapter)
- Referral certification and authorization
- Claims standards
- Claims status
- Payment and remittance advice
- Claims attachments (e.g., medical records and notes)
- Electronic signatures

Electronic billing systems can be utilized with paper charting or with an electronic medical record (EMR) (Figure 12.1). The billing system can be integrated with the EMR or be a separate system.

In a paper record system, in addition to the chart, the physician works with a document called a "superbill" (Figure 12.2). This is an individualized listing of the most commonly performed procedures, office codes, and diagnoses for that physician, department, or office. Usually the provider's name, address, and tax identification number are preprinted on this form. A summary of patient information is filled out by a staff member—name, chart number, birthdate, Social Security number, date of service, insurance company. Modifications and additional codes and diagnoses can be entered in the blank spaces provided. To do this, the physician must memorize the codes or consult a reference book. A copy of the superbill may be given to the patient. The original goes to the billing office where it is entered into the billing system and processed either manually or electronically, depending on the office setup.

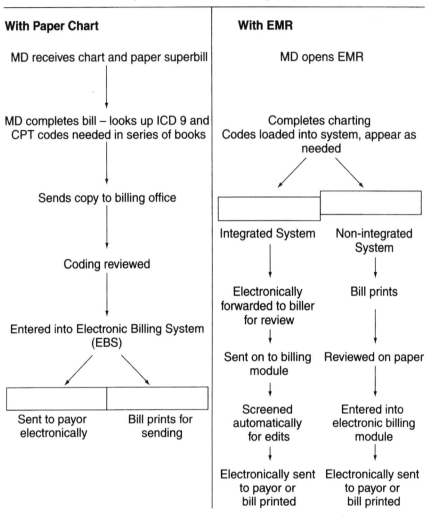

Options for Electronic Billing (EB)

With Paper Chart

MD receives chart and paper superbill

↓

MD completes bill – looks up ICD 9 and CPT codes needed in series of books

↓

Sends copy to billing office

↓

Coding reviewed

↓

Entered into Electronic Billing System (EBS)

Sent to payor electronically | Bill prints for sending

With EMR

MD opens EMR

Completes charting
Codes loaded into system, appear as needed

Integrated System | Non-integrated System

↓ | ↓

Electronically forwarded to biller for review | Bill prints

↓ | ↓

Sent on to billing module | Reviewed on paper

↓ | ↓

Screened automatically for edits | Entered into electronic billing module

↓ | ↓

Electronically sent to payor or bill printed | Electronically sent to payor or bill printed

FIGURE 12.1. Steps for electronic billing (EB) starting with a paper chart or an electronic medical record (EMR).

In an electronic medical record (EMR) (see Chapter 2), the billing may be done on the computer system, where the appropriate codes and diagnoses can be looked up using preset preferred code lists, searches, and pattern matching. Codes can be associated with specific procedures and/or modifiers (Figure 12.3).

If the practice has an interfaced or integrated billing module, the bill is then sent via computer to the billing office for review and forwarding to the payer, usually electronically. If the EMR is not associated with a billing module, the bill is printed and handled as in a paper setting.

In the current era, certain billable items require different coding depending on insurer and circumstance, and thus a stop in the billing office to ensure compli-

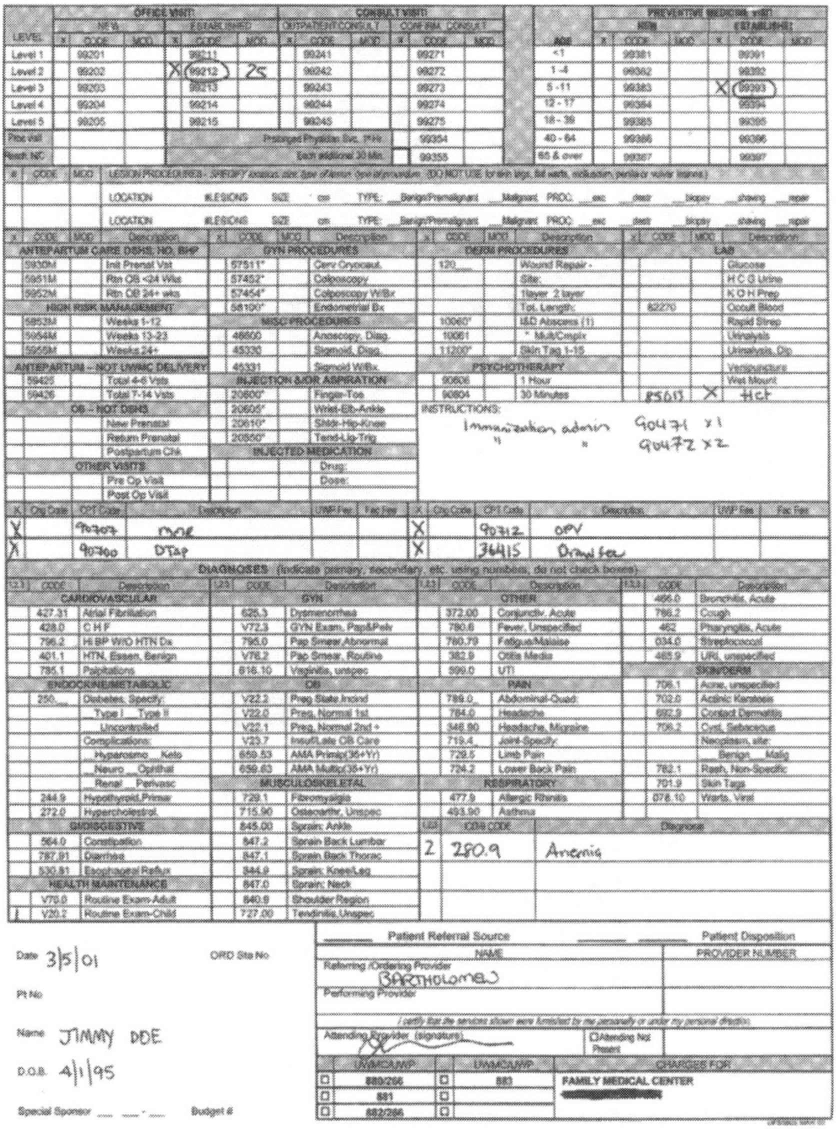

Figure 12.2. A superbill is an individualized listing of the most commonly performed procedures, office codes, and diagnoses used by a physician, department, or office.

ance is a necessity, regardless of the system used. However, the electronic billing system can be set to make certain changes automatically and can also be programmed to edit out claims of a given nature for special review.

Before the patient visit, the office staff can collect certain nonmedical information from the patient in person, by phone, or via patient data entry at a Web portal or via e-mail. Key information that must be collected and entered on billing forms for all patients:

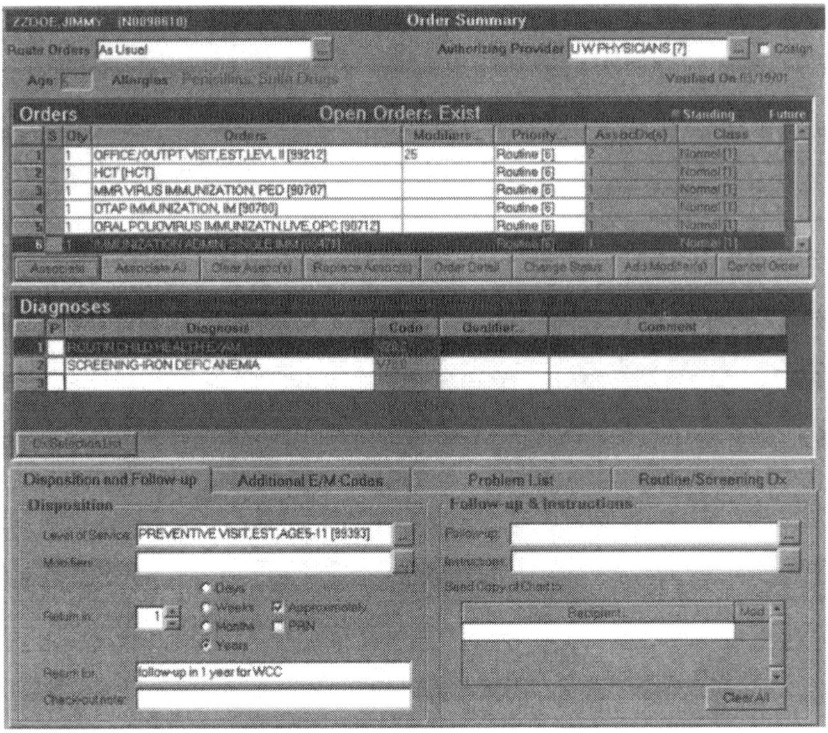

FIGURE 12.3. In an electronic medical record (EMR), the bill may be prepared on a computer system.

• Name of the patient
• Social Security number
• Birth date
• Zip code of patient's residence
• Insurance information: Name of insurance company, plan number, name of insured, insured's identification number

During the patient encounter, the doctor (or staff) must assign a service code to the care received by the patient. These are the five-digit current procedural terminology (CPT) codes, published by the American Medical Association (AMA). The most common code for a primary care physician is 99213 (follow-up visit). Third-party payers will reimburse only for certain codes, and there may be legal issues for them as to whether or not they can reveal the codes before receiving a billing. One of the prime management skills in today's reimbursement environment is to know which codes will be accepted by which payers. To further complicate things, third-party payers (especially private insurance companies) regularly change the CPT codes that they will accept.

The financial viability of a primary care practice depends on using the correct billing codes. Errors in coding slow the speed with which providers are paid. Errors that are easily detected by the insurance companies or public payers result in billings being returned unpaid. Delays in preparation of correct billings are to the advantage of the third-party payers, so a primary care practice can expect little help from those paying the bills.

During or following the patient encounter, the physician must also make a diagnosis and assign it one of the codes from the International Classification of Diseases (ICDA) listings. The diagnosis drives the amount that some payers (e.g., Medicare) pay for the care that the patient receives. Currently the push is on for five-digit billing—the three-digit code and a two-digit "specifier." Frequently payers will "downcode" or reject altogether payments for visits that are given nonspecific diagnoses. It is anticipated that even higher levels of specificity will be required in the future. In addition to the five-digit code, right, left, and bilateral modifiers are already being requested even for nonsurgical visits. An EMR/electronic billing system can help ensure proper coding by making available only the specified codes for given diagnoses.

In a paper setting, the provider must give the superbill to a billing clerk who then looks up the charges in a price master if a patient chooses to pay on the day of service. This assumes that the price master being used is the most recent one. If a billing service is used, the patient may need to call another office altogether. The process is similar in an unintegrated EMR setting. If the office has an integrated system, then the balance due based on the latest price master is available as soon as the provider enters the charges into the record. Other details of the patient's account are also readily available to anyone with appropriate security access.

The insurance companies then sort and process the claims based on the system to detect various problems—cancelled insurance, incorrect patient information, unusual or possibly inappropriate charges—and renders a payment and/or an explanation of benefits (EOB) sheet to both the patient and the provider. The EOB indicates which charges were paid at what rates and why and shows the outstanding patient balance. The provider then bills the remainder to the patient on a patient statement. The provider and/or the patient can choose to challenge the result, and a review process can be started in motion.

Sometimes the payer notifies the provider that payment is pending a review of the records. The appropriate records are submitted with appropriate reference numbers through the mail (for now). An interesting system oddity is that switching to paper and sending the notes with the bill on paper as an initial move does not always speed up the payment process due to insurance workflows. For example, with some payers it is faster to submit an electronic claim, obtain a claim number, and then submit the chart notes. The payer then refers these to the EB and pays the claim; paper bills sit for several weeks longer awaiting manual processing, even if all the information is all together in one place. Billings with missing information are returned to the practice submitting the bill.

In sum, the following must be submitted for every patient.

- CPT service code
- ICDA diagnosis code
- Social Security number
- Birthdate
- Zip code of patient
- Name of insurance company
- Plan number
- Name of insured
- Insured's identification number

How Does Electronic Billing Coordinate with Other Aspects of Modern Practice?

An integrated electronic billing system can be critical to the healthy functioning of a medical office. Copay collection, assignment of payer, data collection, and payment review are all speeded by EB. Patients can have multiple account payers depending on the visit—a personal account (or two if a spouse or parent has additional insurance to cover the patient), an occupational medicine account, a DLI (Department of Labor & Industries) account, an MVA (Motor Vehicle Accident) account, and a separate mental health coverage account. EB can help keep claims on the way to the correct payer. EB can sort bills in a variety of ways to ease payment review and specialized billing practices needed for the various payers. The EB database can be searched for coding and QA reviews. If integrated with an EMR, EB can reduce compliance concerns by ensuring that all claims are tied closely with the appropriate documentation.

Who Uses Electronic Billing Now?

Electronic billing is prevalent in many types of practices. For example, one solo rural practicioner we contacted estimates that he makes two thirds of his claims electronically. Following is a summary of what is happening with various third-party payers.

- *Medicare* Medicare maintains the standard form for billing (the HCFA 1500) that is used by almost all third-party payers (Figure 12.4). There are both paper and electronic versions of this form. Medicare is run at the federal level by the Health Care Financing Administration (HCFA). Officials in Region 10 (Pacific Northwest states) report that over 80% of their billing activity is electronic. The 20% of the bills that come in on paper are from providers who claim that they are too small or too rural to bill electronically. (Of course, size and rurality have nothing to do these days with ability to bill electronically.)
- *Medicaid* Electronic billing varies from state to state. In addition, most states reimburse for Medicaid on a capitated basis. According to HCFA, as of June 1999 only two states, Alaska and Wyoming, did not have any managed Medic-

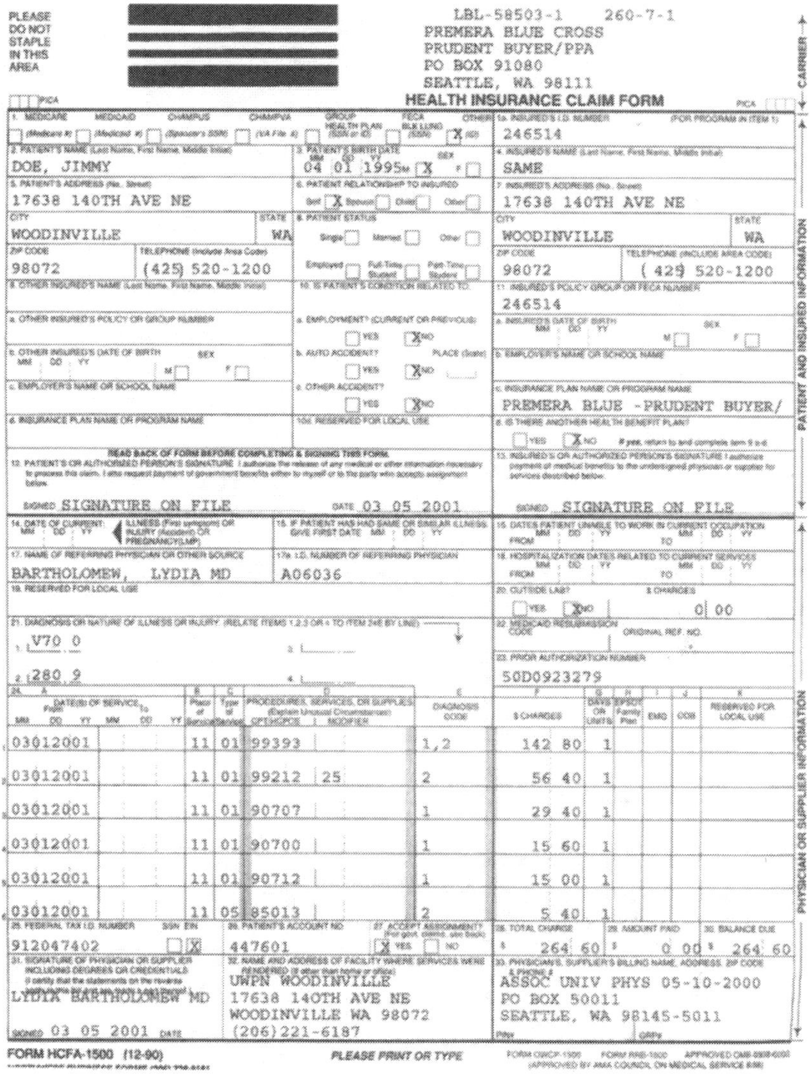
PLEASE DO NOT STAPLE IN THIS AREA

LBL-58503-1 260-7-1
PREMERA BLUE CROSS
PRUDENT BUYER/PPA
PO BOX 91080
SEATTLE, WA 98111

HEALTH INSURANCE CLAIM FORM

1a. INSURED'S I.D. NUMBER: 246514
2. PATIENT'S NAME: DOE, JIMMY
3. PATIENT'S BIRTH DATE: 04 01 1995 SEX: M X
4. INSURED'S NAME: SAME
5. PATIENT'S ADDRESS: 17638 140TH AVE NE
6. PATIENT RELATIONSHIP TO INSURED: Self X
7. INSURED'S ADDRESS: 17638 140TH AVE NE
CITY: WOODINVILLE STATE: WA
CITY: WOODINVILLE STATE: WA
ZIP CODE: 98072 TELEPHONE: (425) 520-1200
ZIP CODE: 98072 TELEPHONE: (425) 520-1200
11. INSURED'S POLICY GROUP OR FECA NUMBER: 246514
10a. EMPLOYMENT? NO X
10b. AUTO ACCIDENT? NO X
10c. OTHER ACCIDENT? NO X
11c. INSURANCE PLAN NAME OR PROGRAM NAME: PREMERA BLUE - PRUDENT BUYER/
11d. IS THERE ANOTHER HEALTH BENEFIT PLAN? NO X

READ BACK OF FORM BEFORE COMPLETING & SIGNING THIS FORM.
12. PATIENT'S OR AUTHORIZED PERSON'S SIGNATURE
SIGNED SIGNATURE ON FILE DATE 03 05 2001
13. INSURED'S OR AUTHORIZED PERSON'S SIGNATURE
SIGNED SIGNATURE ON FILE

17. NAME OF REFERRING PHYSICIAN OR OTHER SOURCE: BARTHOLOMEW, LYDIA MD
17a. I.D. NUMBER OF REFERRING PHYSICIAN: A06036
20. OUTSIDE LAB? NO X $ CHARGES 0 00
21. DIAGNOSIS OR NATURE OF ILLNESS OR INJURY
1. V70 0
2. 280 9
23. PRIOR AUTHORIZATION NUMBER: 50D0923279

24A. Date(s) of Service	B. Place of Service	C. Type of Service	D. CPT/HCPCS	Modifier	E. Diagnosis Code	F. $ Charges	G. Days or Units
03012001	11	01	99393		1,2	142 80	1
03012001	11	01	99212	25	2	56 40	1
03012001	11	01	90707		1	29 40	1
03012001	11	01	90700		1	15 60	1
03012001	11	01	90712		1	15 00	1
03012001	11	05	85013		2	5 40	1

25. FEDERAL TAX I.D. NUMBER: 912047402 EIN X
26. PATIENT'S ACCOUNT NO.: 447601
27. ACCEPT ASSIGNMENT? YES X
28. TOTAL CHARGE: $ 264 60
29. AMOUNT PAID: $ 0 00
30. BALANCE DUE: $ 264 60
31. SIGNATURE OF PHYSICIAN OR SUPPLIER: LYDIA BARTHOLOMEW MD
SIGNED 03 05 2001
32. NAME AND ADDRESS OF FACILITY WHERE SERVICES WERE RENDERED: UWPN WOODINVILLE, 17638 140TH AVE NE, WOODINVILLE WA 98072, (206)221-6187
33. PHYSICIAN'S, SUPPLIER'S BILLING NAME, ADDRESS, ZIP CODE & PHONE #: ASSOC UNIV PHYS 05-10-2000, PO BOX 50011, SEATTLE, WA 98145-5011

FORM HCFA-1500 (12-90) PLEASE PRINT OR TYPE

FIGURE 12.4. HCFA-1500 is a standard form used by most third-party payers.

aid patients. Some states, Tennessee and Washington among them, were at or near 100% managed Medicaid.

- *Commercial insurance companies* Private insurers report lower levels of electronic billing than the 80% cited by HCFA.

Infrastructure Needs in the Provider's Office

Most EB systems work on a standard desktop PC with a modem. Some payers work via the Internet while others have dial-up services. A high-speed connection

TABLE 12.1 Transmission speeds for some common connection options, February 2001.

Terminology	Speed	Multiple of POTS
Plain old telephone service (POTS)	28 Kb–56 Kb	1
Switched 56	56 Kb	1–2
ISDN	128 Kb per line	2–4
DSL	256 Kb–720 Kb	10–25
Cable modem	128 Kb–1 Mb	5–36
T-1	1.45 Mb	50
Ethernet	>10 Mb	>350
Fiber optics	>100 Mb	>3,500

(like DSL or a cable modem) is an advantage but not necessary. Suffice it to say, however, that the need for speed of transmission will probably double every few years (Table 12.1).

EB software can cost from $5,000 to $6,000 for a simple system to hundreds of thousands of dollars for a full-service office management package. This places the small-volume primary care physician (PCP) in a dilemma: she wants to be able to participate in EB but cannot afford a full-service package that has unneeded capabilities.

The staff in the PCP's office must be trained and comfortable with computer applications. Most vendors of EB services provide training for the office staff. Training of providers can be a significant barrier in many places.

Other Aspects

As noted, the EMR can integrate with the EB to form a seamless unit providing large amounts of useful data and improving patient satisfaction with the billing process.

EB can be used to carefully track utilization. This assists internally with planning and contract negotiations and allows a comparison to be made with data from the HMO. Furthermore, this information can be used to satisfy contractually required utilization review. It can also be used to provide data to providers regarding targets for utilization, prevention, and other services.

Sometimes EB companies will also do credit and collections for client practices, but there are laws against it in some states. There are also issues around what information (e.g., credit information and social security information) is legal to send an insurance company.

What Are the Strategic Aspects of EB for Providers?

Table 12.2 summarizes the advantages and disadvantages of electronic billing.

TABLE 12.2 Advantages and disadvantages of electronic billing.

Advantages	Disadvantages
Reduced accounts receivable	Costly equipment purchases
Lower practice costs	Overreliance on automation
Increased business information	Loss of control by the clinician
System efficiency	Nonstandardization of remittances

Advantages

Reduced Accounts Receivable (AR). It is good business to do everything possible to reduce the amount of time it takes to get paid for services provided, and clearly electronic billing is one such mechanism. "Days in AR" is a critical business monitor. EB allows claims to be sent out more quickly and cleanly, reducing the turnaround time and thus the AR. This provides an inflow of cash to the business. Some third parties make payments to providers electronically. Even payers like Medicare that deliberately sit on claims for several weeks before processing them end up with shorter payment intervals because there is much less paperwork at each end of the transaction. In addition, some payers provide financial incentives to bill electronically. Finally, EB systems (whether office-based or at a clearinghouse) have electronic filters that catch billing errors before they go out the door. Errors caught early can save weeks in terms of getting reimbursement.

Lower Practice Costs. Whether bills are done on paper or by modem, the same information gets keyed into a form by the physician's office. To prepare a traditional paper bill, the physician must purchase paper and a printer. There are also the costs of mailing the claims and the expenses of handling and filing the hard copies of claims submitted. The payer too incurs costs in handling the paper and also probably has to reenter the data into its computer system. Claims can only be manually reviewed, and at each data entry point there is room for error. Users of electronic billing believe that they have fewer billing errors because the bills can be edited automatically as well as manually and because there are fewer manual data entry points. Additionally there appear to be fewer lost claims, again due to less handling.

Increased Business Information. Some payers send explanations of benefits on various patients via the electronic billing mechanism. In addition, some payers also send coordination of benefits (secondary insurance) information to providers, helping them work with patients for claims payment.

System Efficiency. When a PCP uses an EB system, the office is the only place the information has to be keyed in. The third-party payer benefits from not having to repeat the keyboard work and having no paper to deal with and can pass some of those savings on to patients and PCPs. If there is an integrated EMR system, information is keyed in as part of the office visit, and another step is saved. All trends show a future with the electronic medical record as the single entry point for all management and financial information; the number of resources currently devoted in the practice of medicine to managing information necessary to get clinicians paid is simply staggering.

Disadvantages

EB does have a few disadvantages.

Cost of Gearing Up. Setting up an EB system and getting it to work properly can take months. As one provider says, "Getting the bugs out took 6 months, and that was a pain and a headache. But once you have it, you cannot live without it." The new Web-based systems, once they pass the start-up hurdles, may provide a lower-cost alternative.

Assuming that the Practice Is Now Fully Automated. While EB can assist in making the billing process simpler, more accurate, and less time consuming, it cannot completely replace the judgment and skill of the office staff. Even with EB as an imbedded system in a comprehensive office management software package (like Medical Manager), the practice still has a lot to do. On the front end, correct coding by the provider is essential to obtaining appropriate reimbursement. The system can load the codes, but the provider must know what codes are available and how and when to use them. On the back end, claims editing can be only partially automated due to the nature of the work. Payer appeals and payment review require staff with specific skill sets. AR monitoring and the development of adequate and timely collection procedures to ensure payment also require personal intervention.

Loss of Control. Once billings go to a clearinghouse, the primary care provider needs to make sure that she gets a report giving assurances that the billing was handled correctly. Disallowed claims must be itemized to give the primary care provider a chance to change the billings or to pursue payment from the patients. This activity requires skill, time, and diligence that a small practice may be unable to afford.

Nonstandardization of Remittances. Although primary care providers are required to standardize their claims submittals (via the HCFA 1500), payers are not similarly required to make remittances to primary care providers in a standard format. This makes the job in the primary care provider's office of receiving remittance reports from the third-party payer an important and difficult management task.

What Does the Future Hold for Electronic Billing?

It does not appear at this time that PCPs will be required to use EB in the near future. But as standardization is implemented, providers will find more and cheaper tools available.

There is great potential for cost savings via Web-based EB functions, but at this writing there is little activity in this area. One possibility is that a provider could, via the Internet, gain access to an insurer's internet. This would allow real-time monitoring of the progress of bills through the insurer's processing. Key concerns will be privacy, security, and encryption.

Physicians and the national associations will be key in implementing standards to make the tie-in of EB to EMR work. Healtheon Web MD is a large national clearinghouse working on changes in the EMR to make it friendly from the physician's point of view.

The Health Insurance Portability and Accountability Act of 1996 (HIPAA) administrative simplification will be a big factor when the act is ultimately implemented. The final rules have been set and large insurers must comply by October 2002. They will be forced to generate and process standard transactions, so this will help EB. Concerns remain over privacy; unique, permanent national identification numbers for providers and patients that are retired when the provider or patient dies will be necessary.

HIPAA will also mandate standard billing forms. The new Accredited National Standard Institute (ANSI) data submission forms have 1,500 data fields, a substantial increase over the current proprietary forms now in use. This would allow providers to weave practice management information into their billing systems (e.g., patient weight, National Drug Codes, and so on).

Some payers (e.g., Medicare) already accept only EB, and some other third-party payers remit funds and itemized statements to PCP electronically. Soon this will be true for all third-party payers. Although this step clearly is coming, it will increase the complexity of billing in the PCP office. Although it is tedious to post all payments (from insurers) manually to the practice's accounting system, the current system is fairly easy to control. Once information and funds start coming back electronically, the danger of systematic (and perhaps disastrous) errors increases. The complexities and uncertainties mean that humans will always have jobs in billing offices, no matter how high-tech they become.

How Do You Get Started if You Do Not Already Do Electronic Billing?

First you must decide the scope of the endeavor. Stand-alone or off-site billing? Integrated with EMR or separate? Generally the size of the practice and the budget dictate some of these choices. As with any investment, a good review of the costs and benefits and a mini business plan are good ideas.

The office practice that wants to "get on line" and start participating in EB needs to be careful in seeking help. There are hundreds of individuals and groups offering to set up EB for primary care physicians. A quick look at the *Wall Street Journal* reveals many EB services that are new businesses with little real-world experience. The doctor who purchases help with EB needs to look beyond just price and find a provider with a track record of success. Low-cost consultants who make mistakes out of inexperience can cost their clients money through delayed claims payments and lost charges. Inexperienced providers also might not know the criteria used by each insurance company and/or might not be able to do EB with all third-party payers. Several payers have banded together to look for ways to standardize the process.

A good strategy for making the EB decision is to hire an outside consultant to help you find an EB company. The consultant will be objective and have only the incentive to help you find a competent service. The PCP could do this search, but his or her primary value to the practice is being a physician and generating patient visits.

If you are considering hiring an EB company, here is a checklist of things to ask. From the checklist, you can develop a scoring sheet.

• Names of references
• Current client list
• Sites we can visit.

When visiting a site ask:

• If money were not an issue, would you go with this system again?
• How often is the system down?
• What is longest it has ever been down?
• What happens when it is down?
• How many third-party payers do you help us work with?
• What are all of the costs of the system/service?
• Can you do a demonstration of the system for us?
• What assurances can you give that our system will remain functional even if there are big changes in the industry? (e.g., web-based billing, new laws like HIPAA, etc.)

Readings and resources

The National Library of Medicine (http://www.nlm.nih.gov) has databases that will produce citations concerning electronic billing. Given the rapid change in this arena, the reader is advised to visit this site for the most current articles on the subject. Medline/PubMed, available free from the NLM website, is a particularly useful database. The following terms could be used for searching for current articles on electronic billing: Insurance Claim Reporting; Medical Records Systems, Computerized; Office Automation; Practice Management, Medical.

Steven Kriebel, M.D., private physician in Forks, Washington
Ron Rehn, Practice Manager, HEW Medical Group, Colville, Washington
Linda Frinberg, Owner, The Medical Office Connection, medicaloffice.com, Seattle, Washington
David Berk, health services financial consultant, Anacortes, Washington
David Masuda, M.D., Department of Health Services, University of Washington School of Public Health
Martin Strand, Manager Electronic Data Interchange manager, Premera Blue Cross of Washington and Blue Cross Blue Shield of Alaska, Mountlake terrace, Washington

13
Reporting and Analysis

P. Jeffrey Hummel, M.D., M.P.H., and
Teresa A. Spellman Gamble, M.P.A.

Scenario 1

You are the director of clinical quality for primary care in an integrated delivery system with 10 primary care clinics, which use a networked electronic medical record (EMR). For the second time this month you have received a phone call from the chairman of the anesthesiology department complaining about the quality of presurgical evaluations done in your department. This time a patient referred for elective surgery by one of your physicians was discovered to have a history of a myocardial infarction by a nurse in the anesthesiology department just before going into the operating room. This cardiac history was not reflected in the patient's problem list and is not mentioned in the preop exam write-up. As a result the surgery was cancelled and the patient was referred to a cardiologist. You decide to bring this incident to the Quality Improvement Committee for review not as a reprimand but as a quality improvement project.

1. What are the problems pertaining to clinical quality in this case?
2. How might the electronic medical record be used to improve quality in preoperative assessment?
3. What is the role of clinical reporting in solving this problem?
4. How would we know that an improvement has taken place?

Scenario 2

The physicians in your network are complaining that the EMR has increased their workload and reduced their productivity. They have cited as an example the management of patients taking warfarin. With the paper chart used in the past, a nurse maintained a three-ring binder with a page for each patient on warfarin. On this page was a graph on which was charted the INR and the dose of warfarin each time the prothrombin time was tested. The nurse would review the binder once a week and call patients for whom testing was due and, when necessary, change the warfarin dose after consulting with the physician. Now the only nurses in the organization are working as telephone consultants in a centralized location. The results of all INRs come back to each physician in their results in-basket on the computer screen. It is the responsibility of the physician to decide whether or not the dose of warfarin needs to be changed and to create a future-dated electronic reminder to the medical assistant to call the patient to come for repeat prothrombin time testing.

1. How might the electronic medical record be used to track a large group of patients taking warfarin rather than simply responding to the needs of one patient at a time?
2. Is managing warfarin an efficient use of the physician's time? If so, is there a way to be reimbursed for it? If not, which nonphysicians should be doing this work and what changes in workflow process might physicians see as an improvement?
3. What kind of clinical reports would assist the person who is doing this work?
4. What are the best ways to identify quality problems with anticoagulation therapy and to determine whether or not quality is improving?

Introduction and Overview

One of the ongoing challenges that healthcare professionals face is sifting through and interpreting the vast amount of data and separating what is relevant from what is irrelevant in planing a course of action. In primary care, this activity takes place every day. An internist might review a patient's EKG readings, vital signs, lab results, and symptoms and, based on her interpretation of the information, choose a course of action that will ultimately have an impact on the patient's opportunity for improved health. This task of interpreting data becomes much more complicated when the internist wants to look at her entire practice, as described in the introductory scenarios.

A distinction must be made between data and information. Data are the abstract representations of things, facts, concepts, and instructions stored in a defined format and structure on a passive medium (paper, computer disk, database). Information is obtained when data are translated into results and statements useful for decision making.

"Data refers to raw facts and figures which are collected as part of the normal functioning of the hospital. Information, on the other hand, is defined as data which have been processed and analyzed in a formal, intelligent way, so that the results are directly useful."[1]

"Data will never become information unless your problem or question is very clearly defined," says John F. Grabowski, researcher/planner for Wausau Hospital in Wisconsin.[2] Data can be produced by pushing a button on a computer or by entering lab results in a patient's chart. Information is produced when the right question is asked (e.g., How has this patient's TSH level changed over the last 12 months?) and the data are analyzed to provide the answer.

The process required to manually combine and aggregate data is time and resource intensive in the paper medical record world, relatively straightforward in the electronic environment. Via the use of data warehouses and applications software, data from an EMR system can be merged with data from financial and other databases and translated into information for clinical improvement as well as practice management and service quality improvement. Data warehouse technology is a crucial supporting technology for EMR systems, as it provides an easily accessible, complete, and reliable source of information that helps to integrate all the care modalities.[3]

The increased availability of data through information technology provides tremendous potential for health care improvement; however, it is the reporting, analysis, and ultimate interpretation of data that give them life. Via the improved accessibility and reliability of data in the primary care informatics environment, integrated information can be reported and analyzed regularly and displayed in a format that is easily understood.

Data Collection Principles

Data can be classified as being one of three types: measurement, count, or subjective.

Measurement data yield a number for each observation or unit and can be subdivided often indefinitely. Measurement data are also called variable, analog, or continuous data. Examples are weight, temperature, time, and cost.

Count data consist of counts of observations or incidents falling into categories; count data is also referred to as discrete, attribute, or digital data. Examples are appointment no-show rates, daily office visits, and number of injuries.

Example: Measuring how long it takes to receive a lab result and plotting each time a result is received is using measurement data—each lab result becomes one data point. When counting the total number of lab results received within 24 hours, the total received within a week, and the total received in more than 7 days, only one data point is gathered for each interval. These data points are described as count data. Generally speaking, information conveyed showing measurement data is much richer than reports of count data.

Quality is often measured by using subjective data, that is, the patient's perception of or reactions to a process, product, or service, gathered by using a questionnaire with subjective rating scales (e.g., Good, Very good, Satisfied, Somewhat satisfied). Even though data are subjective and perhaps imprecise, they can be valuable for understanding key quality characteristics—which are subjective. Functional status and health-related quality of life scores allow assessment of the impact of sickness or a medical intervention on the basic health-related functions of life.

Defining Measures/Indicators

One of the critical issues in reporting and analysis is whether the right data are measured or counted for the right purpose. Indicators, or performance measures, must be clearly defined to ensure the reliability and consistency of the measurement (Table 13.1). Operational definitions help to articulate what is being measured. The operational definition includes three components: the measure, the

TABLE 13.1 Performance indicator criteria

Validity	Must measure what it is supposed to measure.
Reliability	A reliable metric measures the attribute consistently over time
	Development of operational definitions provides the foundation for validity and reliability of measures.
Accuracy	An accurate measure can be verified.
	The methods by which data are collected drive data accuracy.
Timeliness	Real-time performance improvement cannot meet its goals when the data it relies on are not timely.
Relevance	Relevant to the organization.
	Reflects the major business strategy goals and objectives and quantifies the progress made toward meeting them.
	Measures and data must also matter to the customer.
Precise definitions	Measure should have a clear, written definition that is not subject to different interpretations.
	If it is a rate-based indicator, the numerator and denominator must be clearly defined.
Sensitivity	Must be sensitive enough to discern changes in the attribute it is measuring.
Feasibility	Collection must be possible.
Ease of understanding	Must be simple and easy to understand.

Source: Gilbreath E., Schilp JL. *Health Data Quest*. How to find and use Data for Performance Improvement. San Francisco: Jossey Bass, 2000.

instrument to be used in measuring, and the procedure for measuring. It is vital that each of these components be clearly defined, understood, and consistently used by all data analysts.

By conducting the data analysis and reporting electronically, many performance criteria become inherent in the process. Data collected electronically, for example, are more reliable and accurate than data that are manually collected because the process can be automated. In addition, information can be reported in a very timely fashion when the human factor—manual tracking and collecting—is removed. And with a fully functioning informatics environment, collecting data on an ongoing basis is efficient, cost effective, and feasible.

A number of different types of indicators may be used for healthcare improvement: administrative and financial measures and measures of clinical performance, health status, service and satisfaction. Each can be reported at different levels of detail—by patient, physician, condition, procedure, and so on. The table in Table 13.1A outlines some of the indicators used on the fictitious Green Valley primary care provider monthly report. The table identifies each measure, the overall concept it is articulating, the operational definition, the source of the data, and the collection mechanisms. By spelling out these components of performance measures, the reliability and consistency of the measurement is ensured.

Sources of Data

Data collection can be both expensive and time consuming in the paper environment. In the fully functioning computerized clinical environment, accessing data

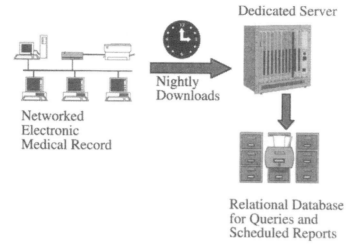

FIGURE 13.1. A networked EMR and relational database.

can be a much more automated process. However, the presence of data in a computerized medical record does not mean that the data are automatically available in a format that can be used to provide useful information in a report.

An electronic medical record in normal operation is perpetually in motion and constantly changing. During the day clinical data are added continuously by providers and staff, while at night data are entered by automated entry of laboratory results and accessing the system from home by providers on call. Before clinical data from patient visits, laboratory results, and pharmacy can be used for any kind of reporting, they must be downloaded into a static form as a relational database, as shown in Figure 13.1. The relational database must be constructed with defined data fields to contain each specific data type that will be used in the reports. One such data field, for example, would contain the date of the most recent blood pressure, while another would hold the diastolic blood pressure value that was recorded on that date. Each selected data type in the EMR is routed to the appropriate data field. Downloads of data can be scheduled to occur nightly so that the data for any given report are never more than 24 hours old. The interface for this kind of download can be a challenge to maintain as software programs are upgraded, laboratories make changes in their tests, and medications are added to or deleted from a formulary[4] (see also Chapter 3).

Translating Data into Meaningful Information

Integrated performance data must be shared with clinicians to determine opportunities for improvement, to benchmark or compare their performance to that of others, and to assess their performance on key aspects of patient care. Data may relate to services provided in the primary care physician's office, referrals to spe-

TABLE 13.1A Green Valley Clinics—Primary Care Provider Instrument Panel Data Collection Plan (EXCERPTS FROM PLAN).
A monthly report of individual Green Valley primary care provider activity, with detailed information as noted below:

Specific Measure	Key Concept	Operational Definition	Data Source	Collection/Collaboration: • Schedule • Method • Responsibility
Total New Patients	Practice Growth	All provider encounters in departments 100–199 (Green Valley) with CPT codes where level of service (LOS) = 99435, 99431, and all codes starting with 9920X and 9938X.	Epic > Clarity > Crystal Reports	Clarity report from IS automatically generated on the 10th day of each month. Email sent to QI Department with reports as attachments.
Total Encounters	Practice Productivity/Growth	All provider encounters* in departments 100–199 (Green Valley) *including* Global Procedures and *excluding* 'opened in error', 'noch' no charge codes, blank procedure codes and codes 2001, 2002, and 2003. *All encounters includes: 99202, 99203, 99204, 99205, 99212, 99213, 99214, 99215, 99385, 99386, 99395, 99396, 99397. A quarterly recount is done to account for visits in which coding was delayed resulting in a 2–3% increase.	Epic > Clarity > Crystal Reports	Clarity report from IS automatically generated on the 10th day of each month. Email sent to QI Department with reports as attachments.
Provider MGMA Benchmark Encounters	Practice Productivity Benchmark	Total Monthly Median Encounters Benchmark number by Specialty adjusted for Provider Clinical FTE • Family Practice with OB (383) • Internal Medicine (336) • Pediatrics (414) • PA-C, ARNP (291)	Based on the annual benchmark from the Medical Group Management Association's (MGMA) 1999 Survey of physician/midlevel compensation and productivity based on 1998 data, Table 36 (Table 92 for PA-C/ARNP) and on the annual benchmark from the MGMA's 1999 Survey of physician compensation and productivity based on 1998 data, Table 44.	Updated annually to reflect changes in MGMA benchmark numbers Text: MGMA Cost Survey Report (Annual)

Metric	Category	Definition	Source	Reporting
Provider MGMA Encounters % Difference	Practice Productivity	Denominator = Provider MGMA Benchmark adjusted for Clinical FTE; Numerator = The difference between the MGMA Benchmark for a given Provider and the Total Encounters for that Provider	Same as above (MGMA)	Updated annually to reflect changes in MGMA benchmark numbers; Text: MGMA Cost Survey Report (Annual)
Current Month % Appointments Filled	Practice Productivity	Denominator = Total Templated Appointment Minutes Available for patient visits*; Numerator = Total Appointment Minutes Scheduled with Patient Visits*; *Counts MINUTES not time slots. EXCLUDES: (automatically subtracts): Overbooks, Cancellations; INCLUDES: Overrides (as of April 2000) and No Shows	Variation of a standard Cadence Report. Combines reports of all providers.	Appointment Scheduling (VFD, PSRs); IS: Cadence Report sent to QI via e-mail on the 7th day of each month; QI: MS Excel Calculation
Current Month No Shows	Clinic Operations	Percent of patients by provider who do not show for scheduled visit appointments (Scheduled Appointment Changed to "No Show"); Denominator = Total number of visits by provider; Numerator = Number of patients who no show for a visit by provider	Cadence > Clarity > Crystal Reports > Excel	Clinic Staff/Providers; IS report automatically generated on the 10th day of each month
Current Month Average Patient Wait Time	Clinic Operations	The number of minutes a patient waits **from** either 1) appointment time or 2) arrival time (whichever is *later*) **until** the time that the MA selects "Accept" in the Epic Exam screen (usually when vitals are taken). Excludes negative wait times and wait times over 60 minutes.	Cadence > Clarity > Crystal Reports Report EXCLUDES: Residents, RNs, Resources, Dentists. Wait times rounded.	• Appointment time entered in Cadence by TSR; • Arrival time in clinic entered by PSR. (beginning of wait); • Exam opened by MA (end of wait); IS report automatically generated on the 10th day of each month

cialists, laboratory and radiology services, hospital admissions, and prescription drugs.

These data may exist in a variety of source systems, so they must be brought together and reported in an organized manner. The way the information is prepared and presented directly influences the clinicians' willingness to participate in performance improvement opportunities. Providers need and want to see data about their practice, but the news that they are not doing as well as their peers may not always be welcomed. Thus, it is imperative that the information presented is accurate, valid, and reliable. In addition, it must be presented in the most effective and efficient way, helping the clinician to analyze the information quickly.[5]

In translating data into meaningful information, the following questions should be addressed:

• How do these data compare with other organizations' similar data or with previously analyzed internal data?
• What is the trend over time? Is it static, improving, or worsening?
• How are data likely to be interpreted (or misinterpreted)?
• Is there an opportunity for improvement?
• Who should receive this data and for what purpose?

An assortment of analysis and display tools is available to assist with presenting information; tables are the most common form of presentation, though they are not necessarily the most useful. For tables to be their most effective, they should be understandable and utilize minimal abbreviations or jargon. They should have clearly identified columns, and specific findings should be highlighted with boldface type or color. Users should be involved in identifying the measures included on a table to ensure their buy-in and use of the tool.

Graphics and visuals can provide an excellent snapshot of where the practice is, where the variations lie, the relative importance of the identified problems, and the impact, if any, of the changes that have been instituted.[6] Common graphical display techniques include bar charts, histograms, pie charts, and run charts.

Bar Chart

A bar chart is a graphical tool used to display quantitative information about categories of data. Displaying the data in this way allows for comparison of the categories. Bars can be displayed either vertically or horizontally, as in Figure 13.2.

With a bar chart the x-axis consists of discrete categories—each bar is a separate group. Bar charts with a separate bar for each value should be utilized only when data are sparse (<12 values); as the data increases, it becomes necessary to organize and summarize.

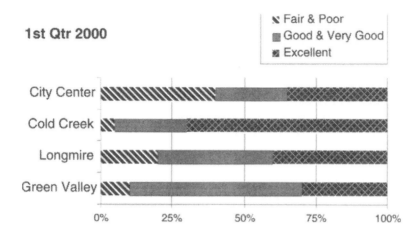

FIGURE 13.2. Results of a patient survey.

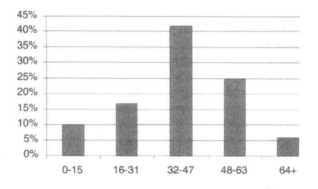

FIGURE 13.3. Age range of Dr. Smith's patients.

Histogram

A histogram is the most commonly used frequency distribution tool. The histogram tells us how a single variable is distributed (what is the spread of Cost, Blood pressure, Age, and so on in our population?). Some other common uses of histograms might be time to complete a type of lab test, minutes waiting time, cost per case, and age.

A histogram graphically displays the distribution of a data set by presenting the measurement scale of values along its x-axis and a frequency scale (as counts or percents) along its y-axis. Plotting the frequency of each interval reveals the pattern of the data showing its center and general distribution (including outliers) and whether there is symmetry or skew. A histogram's x-axis is divided into categories using equal-sized ranges of values along the axis. The variable (age in Figure 13.3) is measured on a continuous scale, and therefore there are no numerical gaps between the bars.

1999 Distribution at Green Valley Clinic

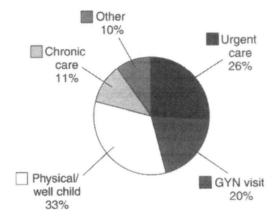

FIGURE 13.4. Distribution of Patient Visit Types.

Pie Chart

A pie chart shows the percentage that each category of values contributes to the total of all values. This is a good basic display technique for communicating distribution within a category, such as patient visit types (Figure 13.4.)

Run Chart

A run chart provides a graphical display of data over time and is one of the tools used to display variation and to detect the presence or absence of special causes. It may also be used to observe the effects of a process improvement experiment. A run chart offers a dynamic display and can be used on virtually any type of data (e.g., counts of events, percentages, and dollars). Most people can easily understand run charts because they require no statistical calculations.[7] A good rule of thumb is to have at least 24 data points on a run chart before using the tests for special cause.

What can be learned from a run chart?

• Baseline performance over time
• Amount/type of variation in process
• If process is changing over time
• If change really was an improvement
• More accurate basis for prediction

The first step in analyzing a run chart is to understand what is meant by a "run." A run is defined as one or more consecutive data points on the same side of the median. In Figure 13.5, the runs range from one data point to three data points, and you can count a total of 15 runs. The purpose of identifying the number of

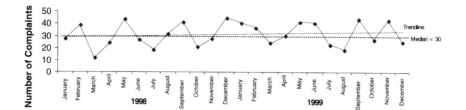

FIGURE 13.5. Patient Complaints Run Chart, 1998–1999.

1998 Complaints		1999 Complaints	
January	28	January	41
February	39	February	37
March	12	March	24
April	24	April	30
May	44	May	42
June	27	June	41
July	19	July	23
August	32	August	19
September	42	September	44
October	21	October	27
November	28	November	43
December	45	December	25
	361		396

FIGURE 13.6. Data from the Patient Complaints Run Chart in Figure 13.5.

runs is to identify whether the process exhibits common or special causes of variation. Three simple tests are applied to the chart to determine the source(s) of the variation:

1. To detect shifts, look for seven or more consecutive points running above or below the median or mean.
2. To detect trends, look for at least six consecutive data points going up or going down.
3. Any nonrandom pattern may indicate a special cause of variation. A general rule is to investigate any nonrandom pattern that recurs seven or more consecutive times.

The run chart in Figure 13.5 tells you that on average, 30 patient complaints are received each month, and the complaints are increasing slightly from last year. No trends, shifts, or patterns are apparent, and thus the process is considered stable.

Compare the run chart to the table in Figure 13.6. Are you able to gain as much information from the table? Trends and shifts in data are much more difficult to discern in tabular format. Those close to the information may be able to identify pat-

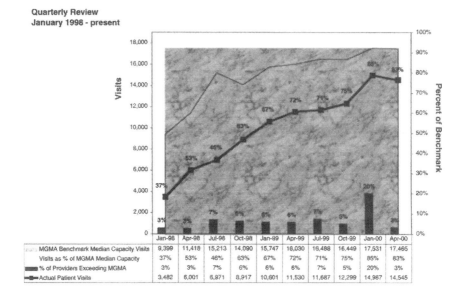

FIGURE 13.7. Growth chart for Green Valley Clinic.

terns, but patterns are not readily apparent to those less familiar with the data. Thus, clinicians are encouraged to use charts and graphs to illustrate and report data.

Another option is to combine a table of data with a graphical representation (Figure 13.7). The reader is able to identify the specific data related to their clinic in the table while gaining a clear understanding of the organizational trends from the graphical display.

Software

No single software application can adequately fill the data analysis, manipulation, and reporting needs of healthcare professionals. In choosing individual software for data analysis and reporting, the following factors should be considered:

• Program capability and versatility: statistical analysis, graphic display, ease of use, and so on
• Integration with existing systems and other software
• Cost

The journal of the American Society for Quality, *Quality Progress,* publishes an annual software directory that describes well over 200 software applications. The directory includes a comparison of cost and program characteristics, as well as contact information for each vendor. Of the vast array available in the market-place, we suggest the following applications:

• A *spreadsheet program* including graphical display, to manage data and assist with calculations. Microsoft Excel is popular.

- A *database management program* to assist in storing and manipulating data. Most have some data analysis capabilities and provide numerous choices in how to sort the data. The most popular relational databases are dBase and Microsoft Access.

Clinical Improvement in Analysis and Reporting: Examples

A clinical practice report is a periodic report that provides information to healthcare providers on outcomes for a group of patients with a specified clinical condition. It is designed to alter clinical outcomes for the group of patients by giving feedback to providers on specific aspects of care related to the desired outcome.[4]

For example, a clinical practice report could be designed to report on the percent of women who have had mammograms to screen for breast cancer within the appropriate time period out of the total population that should receive mammogram screening. To serve the needs of providers the report must be more than a report card. In other words, the report should not only show the provider the percent women who have been screened, it should also include the names of the women who are overdue for a mammogram so that they can be contacted and scheduled for screening, thereby improving the outcome. The goal of the report should therefore be to increase the percent of women who are appropriately screened.[8]

An electronic medical record system provides an opportunity to use the clinical data the records contain for a variety of clinical reports that can be used to guide efforts to track and improve the quality of care patients receive. The development of a useful reporting system, however, is not a simple matter. Reports that are useful to clinicians and serve the purpose for which they were developed require careful teamwork between an organization's leadership, the clinicians who provide care for the patients, and the informatics experts who build the reports. Without collaboration, the result can be reports that are inaccurate, out of date, or irrelevant, leading to frustration for all parties involved.[9]

Clinicians in general are very conscientious and exert tremendous effort to ensure that appropriate diagnostic and treatment interventions are used in their patients' best interests. The value in generating reports for clinical quality lies in three areas.

1. Identifying gaps between providers' beliefs about their outcomes and the measurable outcomes. Reports serve to identify patients who, for a number of reasons, may have fallen through the cracks of a delivery system despite the best efforts of competent clinicians.
2. Identifying of parts of a delivery system that are achieving better clinical outcomes than other parts of the system due to different work processes, which can be replicated to benefit the organization as a whole.
3. Documenting specific outcomes for accreditation and federal oversight agencies and quality assurance entities such as the National Committee for Quality Assurance (NCQA).

Clinical reporting is a tool for improving clinical outcomes. The strategy for improvement in healthcare has been refined in recent years by Nolan and Berwick using an improvement model adapted from other industries. This model consists of four repeating steps in an improvement cycle,[10] as follows:

1. *Plan.* Include definition of the problem and identification of changes in the process of care that might lead to an improvement.
2. *Do.* Carry out small-scale pilot changes in the processes of care.
3. *Study.* Measure the outcomes of the pilot projects to determine whether the changes resulted in an improvement.
4. *Act.* Refine the interventions to improve parts of the new process that could work better. Once the intervention has been sufficiently refined, it can be spread to other parts of the organization.

Reports are crucial in all steps of the improvement cycle.

• Reports provide data to quantify a gap between current outcomes and optimal outcomes according to evidence-based guidelines.
• Reports are used to identify not only patients who have received an intervention but those who have not and for whom the intervention is indicated.
• Once a change has been made in a clinical process, reports provide information to determine whether the change has resulted in an improvement.
• If a new way of providing care can be shown to result in a clinical improvement, reports are used to present the improved outcomes to other parts of a delivery system.

Creating Reports

Building a reporting system in an informatics environment is a complex task that requires a major investment of time and energy. Although reports are easy to run, designing them to give accurate, timely, and reliable information often requires much iteration to find and correct errors. The following steps are important to assure that a reporting project achieves the desired clinical results.

Defining the Problem

A clinical practice report should address a definable and quantifiable gap or deficiency in clinical quality that is deemed important to healthcare providers and their patients. Generally, clinical improvement is measurable as a reduction in morbidity, mortality, or unnecessary cost. The clinical improvement effort should have the support of the organization's leadership. The target clinical issue should have an agreed-on standard of care that is grounded as much as possible in an evidence-based guideline, and it should focus on areas of medicine agreed to be in society's interest.[11]

Defining the Variables

Report designers must solve a number of problems to turn the data in a relational database into a clinically useful report.

Discrimination

The first task in writing a report is to identify a precise way to discriminate between patients to be included in the report and patients to be excluded from the report. The parameters (also called "arguments") used for discrimination will vary depending on the clinical issue the report addresses. The result of the discrimination (selection) process is a list, in the form of a table in the database, containing a unique identifier for each patient (medical history number) to be included in the report. This table forms the basis of a registry by defining the population to which the report pertains, and it serves as the denominator for statistics contained in the report. Patients are added to or removed from the registry depending on whether they meet the criteria in the selection parameters.

1. *Demographic parameters*   A report designed to identify patients in need of a mammogram to screen for breast cancer might start by selecting all female patients over age 50. A lower age threshold can be used for women with additional risk factors such as a family history of breast cancer.
2. *Disease state parameters*   One of the simplest discrimination mechanisms is the presence of a disease-specific ICD-9 code on a patient's problem list. With diabetes, for example, a code between 250.00 and 250.99 on the problem list can be set as a parameter to add a patient's identifier to the disease registry. Arguments can be set to exclude deceased patients and patients whose charts have been inactivated because they have left the system. For this process to work accurately, a secondary report should be created identifying all patients for whom diabetes does not appear on the problem list but who have lab values or are taking medications indicating that they may have diabetes. In this way a nurse can review the chart and make the decision whether or not to add diabetes to the problem list.
3. *Laboratory parameters*   In some cases, there may be no ICD-9 code specific enough to use as a parameter. For example, with chronic infection with a carcinogenic strain of human papilloma virus, there is no code to identify a population of women at risk for cervical cancer.[12] In these cases a laboratory result value entered into the electronic medical record may be used as the selection parameter.
4. *Medication parameters*   Medications may serve as a parameter for identifying patients with a specific condition, provided there are drugs specific to the disease. There are several difficulties inherent in using medications as the discrimination parameter for a population.
   • Many medications, such as beta blockers, are poor markers for a specific disease because they are used for several diseases.
   • Some medications, such as nitroglycerine, H2 blockers or beta agonist-metered dose inhalers, are occasionally prescribed as a therapeutic trial before a clinical diagnosis has been established.
   • Medications often come in many doses, brands, and combinations with other drugs, all of which must be identified if their presence in the chart is to be used as an inclusion parameter.

Henry Higgins, MD
Date of Report: 6/1/01

Name	Identifier	Date Last BP	BP Value
Patient One	N1234567	12/4/00	165/85
Patient Two	N2345678	3/14/01	130/90
Patient Three	N3456789	4/17/01	122/75
Patient Four	N4567890	2/17/98	184/90
Patient Five	N5678901	2/20/01	145/80
Patient Six	N6789012	5/16/01	150/75
Patient Seven	N7890123	4/2/01	130/80
Patient Eight	N8901234	3/21/01	125/79
Patient Nine	N9012345	4/13/01	142/84
Patient Ten	N0123456	5/10/00	150/85

FIGURE 13.8. Clinical practice report on hypertension among patients with diabetes.

- For these reasons the use of medications as disease parameters is often more complex than other discriminators. One exception is when the use of a medication itself rather than the disease for which it is prescribed is the focus of the report. For example, in tracking patients on warfarin, periodic monitoring is required regardless of the reason the medication was prescribed. A report can select all patients with an active prescription for warfarin.
5. *Utilization parameters*   Many diseases, such as asthma, are characterized by a wide variation between patients with very mild, intermittent disease, who may not benefit from disease management, and patients with severe, persistent disease, for whom targeted interventions may improve outcomes. The number of primary care encounters, emergency visits, or hospital admissions within a specified period of time may be used to discriminate between patients.

Data collection

Once the discrimination parameters have been used to populate a registry of all patients with the target condition (denominator), the next step is to define parameters to be used to collect data from the relational database to be included in the report. The data and the parameters chosen for the report are determined by the report's purpose.

In the case of a report on hypertension control among patients with diabetes, a report can be designed to highlight the diabetes patients' systolic and diastolic blood pressure values that are too high. The report would show patients for who the most recent systolic pressure was greater than 130 or the diastolic blood pressure was greater than 85. A second data parameter can be set to highlight the patients whose most recent set of vital signs was more than a year ago. These numbers represent the numerators of the report. The report will then display the names of the patients with diabetes for whom additional intervention (diet, exercise, medication) is required to bring the blood pressure into adequate control by ADA standards as shown in Figure 13.8.

		Date Last A1c	Value
N8196547	PATIENT, ONE	9/27/99 *	▨
N1098765	PATENT, TWO	3/21/00	10.6
N0123456	PATIENT. THREE	4/25/00	7.8
N1357911	PATIENT ,FOUR	6/11/00	▨
N2468100	PATIENT, FIVE	5/14/00	7.9

Number Pts with no recorded HbA1c in last 6mo: 1   **   Total Diabetic Patients
            Percent of Pts overdue for HbA1c: 20.0 %   for Provider   5

Number(%) Pts with last HbA1c for year, <8.0:   2   40.0 %
                          >=8.0-<=9.5:   2   40.0 %
                                >9.5:   1   20.0 %

FIGURE 13.9. A Clinical Practice Report with both process and intermediate outcomes for glycemic control.

The report designers must choose data that are important in managing the target condition. The choice of data to be displayed should, when possible, be founded in evidence-based guidelines and based on the needs of physicians who are the primary audience or customer of the report. Data in reports pertain to either the process or an intermediate outcome of disease management. Both process and intermediate outcome data can be used in the same report, as shown in Figure 13.9.

• *Process data* describe whether or not an action was carried out in the recommended time frame, i.e., whether a test was ordered or a pertinent question was asked. An examples is whether a patient with diabetes had a dilated retinal exam in the last 12 months. If a guideline states that glycosylated hemoglobin should be tested twice a year in all patients with diabetes, a reasonable process measure would give a provider the names of all patients who have not had their HbA1c tested within 6 months. The report should include the date of the most recent test so that its validity can be confirmed by looking in the patient's chart.
• *Intermediate outcome data* reflect actual physiologic variables, such as blood pressure or hemoglobin A1c, which have been clearly associated with long-term health outcomes such as morbidity or mortality. An outcome report may give the provider the names of all patients with diabetes whose most recent total cholesterol HDL ratio is > 4.0. In general, providers have much less control over outcome measures than they do over process measures, since disease severity and comorbidity are major determinants of outcomes.

When designing clinical practice reports it is common to find types of data that should be included in a report but are not available in usable format. For example, a diabetes guideline may call for assessment for peripheral neuropathy by use of a 0.09-mm plastic monofilament for a foot exam at yearly intervals. When the test is performed, the results may simply be entered into the body of a chart note. In this format, it is not possible to query the database to generate a report of all patients overdue for screening or all patients with neuropathy who should receive standardized instructions for self-management of the high-risk diabetic foot.

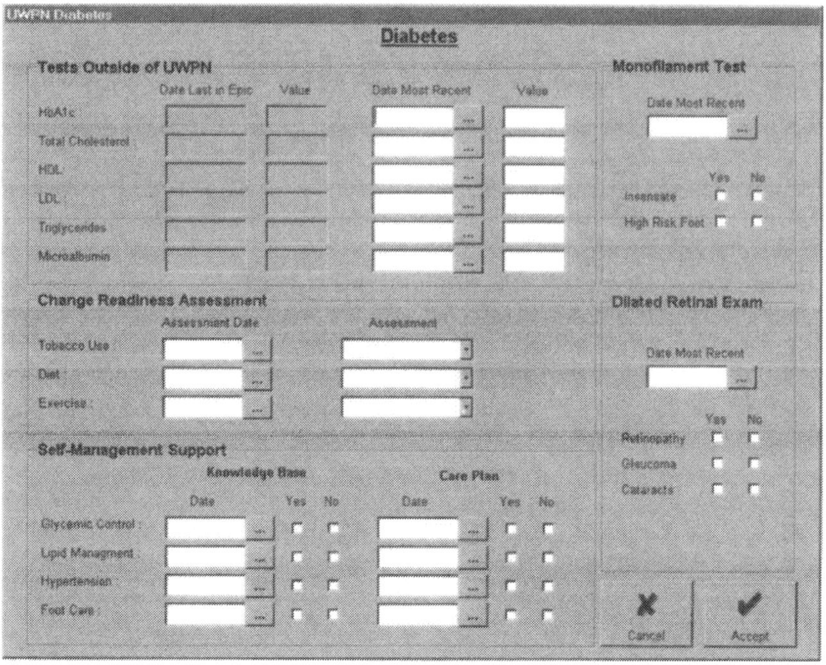

FIGURE 13.10. A supplemental data entry screen for diabetes.

Before data can be included in a report it is necessary to build a data entry. screen into which the data are entered in the electronic medical record and are then stored in discrete data fields. These data can then be made to automatically populate a field in the relational database each time the database is updated. An example of such a data entry screen is shown in Figure 13.10.

Making the Report

The design and layout of a report will depend on the reporting needs of the organization and the capability of the software used to present the data as useful information. In general, the report should display the names of all patients with the target disease. Since providers and chronic illness managers generally know their patients well, they will be the first to identify errors in the report. Patients without the disease who appear on the list and those with the disease who are omitted will serve as a quality check on the many lines of computer code used to generate the registry. For this reason, feedback from providers on the utility of the report is essential. In addition, the ability to see an entire population of patients with a condition such as diabetes or heart failure helps providers develop a population-based perspective on their practice. The names of the patients in need of further interventions are essential for the care team to act on the information in the report.

For the report to be useful in helping plan for resource allocation, providers need to be able to see how they are doing in caring for their patients compared to

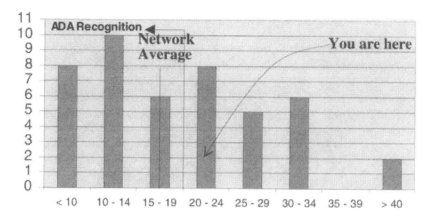

FIGURE 13.11. Histogram of percent diabetic patients with HbA1 > 9.5 by provider.

their peers and compared to a benchmark. A report should display both process and outcome measures as ratios or percents. Comparison data can be displayed for the other providers in the same organization, national benchmarks can be shown, and the report can depict the trend for a provider over time. The histogram in Figure 13.11 shows providers in a primary care network. Each mark on the y-axis represents one provider. The x-axis shows the distribution of providers with different percentages of their patients with diabetes with HbA1c > 9.5. The "You are here" message can be set individually for each provider so that his/her outcome is presented against the data for the organization as a whole and the national benchmark.

Making the Clinician's Job Easier

Clinical practice reports risk being perceived by busy physicians as judgmental meddling by nonclinicians. The best way to avoid this pitfall is for the reports to be designed by physician clinical leaders to achieve better clinical outcomes. The clinical practice report should be part of a disease management program that includes nonphysician clinical team members to carry out the tasks generated by the report (such as calling patients and coaching them in self-management) that will improve the parameters monitored by the report. The report must be seen as a way to help physicians rather than adding work to their busy day.

Putting Theory into Practice

Ambulatory primary care practice is a complex mix of acute care, preventive care, and chronic illness care. Each of these types of primary care work has different reporting needs. The following case studies illustrate some of the challenges inherent in the design of clinical reports in delivery systems using an electronic medical record.

Case Study in Acute Care

Acute care presents a challenge in report writing. Much of acute care involves conditions that are either self-limited or resolved with appropriate treatment over a short period of time. Reports pertaining to diagnosis and therapy for acute care may arrive too late to help the physician improve the care an individual patient receives. The names of the patients are often no longer relevant by the time the report arrives, and feedback may act simply as a report card showing the percent of patients that either did or did not receive a certain standard of care. The effect of the report may be positive feedback for those who have done well; it will be negative feedback for those who may have done poorly without providing clear steps for improving outcomes, since the opportunity for intervention in those patients is past. For our example, we have chosen the situation in which a report is designed to help in the planned care for an acute event in the course of a chronic illness.

Defining the Problem

The hospital anesthesiology department reports that there is a large variation in the primary care preoperative evaluations of patients with known coronary artery disease who are undergoing elective noncardiac surgery. There have been several cases in the past year in which neither the surgeon nor the anesthesiologist realized that a patient had cardiac disease, and one of those patients had postoperative coronary ischemia, which placed the patient at increased risk and resulted in a prolonged hospital stay.

Selecting a Standard of Care

A quality improvement task force is appointed comprising representatives from primary care, cardiology, general surgery, and anesthesiology. After a limited but careful search of the literature on standards for evaluation of cardiac patients before elective surgery, the task force agrees to use a guideline for perioperative cardiovascular evaluation for noncardiac surgery from the American College of Cardiology,[13] shown in Figure 13.2. This guideline stipulates a multistep process for decision making including specifying the urgency of the surgical procedure and whether additional diagnostic testing should be done before surgery for patients with coronary artery disease.

Discrimination: Patient Identification

Patients with coronary disease can be identified with an ICD-9 code 410.0 through 414.9 for coronary artery disease on their problem list. Patients can be added to or deleted from the report by adding or deleting the diagnosis from their problem lists. A table called "CAD," which contains the medical history number of all patients with coronary disease, is then created in the relational database.

Step 1. What is the urgency of noncardiac surgery? Certain emergencies do not allow time for preoperative cardiac evaluation. Postoperative risk stratification may be appropriate for some patients who have not had such an assessment before.

Step 2. Has the patient undergone coronary revascularization in the past 5 years? If so, and if clinical status has remained stable without recurrent symptoms/signs of ischemia, further cardiac testing is generally not necessary.

Step 3. Has the patient had a coronary evaluation in the past 2 years? If coronary risk was adequately assessed and the findings were favorable, it is usually not necessary to repeat testing unless the patient has experienced a change or new symptoms of coronary ischemia since the previous evaluation.

Step 4. Does the patient have an unstable coronary syndrome or a major clinical predictor of risk? When elective noncardiac surgery is being considered, the presence of unstable coronary disease, decompensated CHF, symptomatic arrhythmias, and/or severe valvular heart disease usually leads to cancellation or delay of surgery until the problem has been identified and treated.

Step 5. Does the patient have *intermediate clinical predictors of risk*? The presence or absence of prior MI by history or ECG, angina pectoris, compensated or prior CHF, and/or diabetes mellitus helps further stratify clinical risk for perioperative coronary events. Consideration of *functional capacity* and level of *surgery-specific risk* allows a rational approach to identifying patients most likely to benefit from further noninvasive testing.

Step 6. Patients without major but with intermediate predictors of clinical risk and moderate or excellent functional capacity can generally undergo intermediate-risk surgery with little likelihood of perioperative death or MI. Conversely, further noninvasive testing is often considered for patients with poor functional capacity or moderate functional capacity but higher-risk surgery and especially for patients with two or more intermediate predictors.

Step 7. Noncardiac surgery is generally safe for patients with neither major nor intermediate predictors of clinical risk and moderate or excellent functional capacity (4 METs or greater). Further testing may be considered on an individual basis for patients without clinical markers but poor functional capacity who are facing higher-risk operations, particularly those with several minor clinical predictors of risk who are to undergo vascular surgery.

Step 8. The results of noninvasive testing can be used to determine further preoperative management. Alternatively, the results may lead to a recommendation to proceed with surgery. In some patients, the risk of coronary intervention or corrective cardiac surgery may approach or even exceed the risk of the proposed noncardiac surgery. This approach may be appropriate, however, if it also significantly improves the patient's long-term prognosis.

FIGURE 13.12. The American College of Cardiology algorithm for peri-operative cardiovascular evaluation for noncardiac surgery.

The report designers must also find a way to identify all patients with known coronary disease for which a corresponding ICD-9 code is *not* on the problem list. They create a second report identifying all patients without CAD on the problem list who have been given a encounter diagnosis for coronary ischemia or heart attack in the past or have a past medical history notation for coronary disease. This report lists the patients meeting the above criteria sorted by provider so that charts can be reviewed and the problem lists updated, thereby adding patients to the coronary disease registry.

Assessment	Elective	Urgent	Comments
1. Urgency of surgery:	–	–	
	Yes	**No**	
2. Coronary revascularization within the past 5 years?	–	–	If yes and clinical status is stable without signs of ischemia, further cardiac testing generally not necessary
If so, is clinical status stable?	–	–	
3. Has patient had coronary evaluation in last 2 years?	–	–	If risk was adequately assessed and findings favorable repeat testing usually unnecessary unless changed symptoms.
4. Does patient have unstable coronary syndrome or major predictor of risk?	–	–	Unstable CAD, decompensated CHF, symptomatic arrhythmias, valvular heart disease.
5. Does patient have intermediate clinical predictors of risk?	–	–	Prior MI by hx or EKG, angina, compensated or prior CHF, or diabetes
Decision Making			
6. Patients with intermediate but without major clinical predictors of risk moderate or excellent functional capacity may undergo surgery minimal risk. Consider non-invasive testing for patients with poor to moderate functional capacity or more than one intermediate predictor of risk.			
7. Non-cardiac surgery is generally safe for patients with no major or intermediate predictors of risk. For patients with poor functional capacity facing higher risk surgery, e.g. vascular, consider further testing.			
8. Results of non-invasive testing when necessary should be used to guide preoperative management.			

FIGURE 13.13. Data entry form for pre-operative cardiac assessment for elective surgery.

Data Capture

There are several useful pieces of clinical data in the presurgical cardiac evaluation that could be incorporated into the report. However, the task force decides that the report should not attempt to evaluate the validity of each primary care physician's preoperative assessment. Rather, the report should simply ensure that each patient undergoes an evaluation. The process of evaluation should be standardized to ensure that all providers are using a similar approach without impugning the clinical competence of the physicians. For this reason the task force decides to convert the eight-step evaluation guideline into a data entry form with five yes/no questions and three decision support points for further evaluation, as shown in Figure 13.13.

The CAD presurgical data entry form is designed to appear automatically on the computer screen when patients with coronary artery disease on their problem list are seen for a presurgical exam. Result:

1. A clearly defined process for the primary care providers performing a presurgical evaluation in coronary patients
2. A mechanism for viewing the cardiovascular stability for use by surgeons and anesthesiologists
3. A mechanism for evaluating quality of care

Timeliness of the Report

The clinical value of this reporting system depends primarily on the mechanism for ensuring that coronary disease is on the problem lists of those patients that have it. These patients with coronary disease do not get to surgery without an appropriate cardiac evaluation. Each patient will have the clinical data from the evaluation in their chart at the time of surgery. Per provider, the number of patients with coronary disease who have a presurgical evaluation will be relatively small. For this reason, the task force decides to run the problem list report monthly, while the report on presurgical evaluation can probably be set to run one or two times per year. The report will be most useful in identifying parts of the delivery system in which the standardized approach isn't being used.

Trends in Quality

There are a number of methodological difficulties in comparing outcomes before and after the reporting system is implemented. However, chart reviews can be done to determine the percent of patients with coronary disease in whose charts the illness was not on the problem list prior to implementation of the reporting system. Likewise, chart reviews can determine the approximate percent of patients with coronary disease who underwent elective surgery without adequate evaluation prior to use of the report. Once the reporting system is in use, it will be relatively simple to demonstrate improvement in both these parameters.

Making the Clinician's Job Easier

In addition to the factors mentioned, the report system should make the job of the providers easier by making problem lists on all patients more accurate. Note that someone other than the physicians should probably perform the task of correcting the problem list under the direction of the physician so that this is not perceived as simply one more task for busy providers to do.

Case Study in Chronic Disease Management

Most chronic illnesses, including diabetes, heart failure, HIV/AIDS, and chronic obstructive lung disease, have a relatively stable population, which can be defined by clinical data contained in the medical record. The challenge for chronic illness management is to track a number of variables, such as glycemic control, renal function, or peak expiratory flow rate, over long time intervals.[14] Reporting serves a crucial function in alerting providers or disease managers to patients who are overdue for monitoring, require more aggressive intervention, or have not received training in self-monitoring or behavior modification.

Defining the Problem

A 10-clinic primary care network with an electronic medical record is managing anticoagulation on an ad hoc basis. In most of the clinics, physicians receive the results of the prothrombin times they have ordered as they come in. They adjust the dose of warfarin one patient at a time. A mechanism within each patient's electronic chart reviews the past INRs and finds the dose of warfarin in a flowchart format. A list of all patients on warfarin is maintained. The electronic medical record includes an automated mechanism to notify providers when a patient has not had a prothrombin time within a set time frame, which has been set at 6 weeks for all patients.

The local university wants to train pharmacy residents in the clinics. The pharmacy residents have requested to be allowed to manage the anticoagulation for patients in the network to gain experience with an electronic medical record. This is seen as an opportunity to improve quality by standardizing the process of care while decreasing the workload of individual primary care physicians.[15]

Selecting the Standard of Care

Three parameters determine the care plan for a patient on warfarin. One is the target level of anticoagulation, the second is the interval at which the INR is to be monitored, and the third is length of therapy. The challenge for the developers of this program is that the standards for each of these parameters may vary both between patients and also for the same patient at different points in the treatment. It would be ideal if rather than being held to a single standard for all patients, physicians could determine for each patient what they want the target INR, duration of therapy, and frequency of monitoring to be. The program developers decide to provide on-line decision support for providers for target INR range and duration of therapy based on indication and frequency of monitoring based on clinical context. They will create a data entry screen so that the treatment plan criteria (target INR, monitoring interval, and treatment duration) can be entered into each patient's chart in a form that will be part of the database. The patients own individual treatment plan will be the standard against which the clinical care of the patient is compared. Three reports can then be created to generate lists identifying (1) all patients whose INR is outside of the target range, (2) patients who are still on warfarin after the date that it was to be stopped has passed, and (3) patients who have not had their prothrombin time tested in the desired interval.

Discrimination

There is no ICD-9 code for patients taking warfarin, and in each of the conditions for which warfarin may be used, the decision to anticoagulate is a complex balance of risks and benefits. The report designers decide to use a current prescription for warfarin as their criterion for selection. This means that patients will show up on the report if the chart indicates they are still taking warfarin even if they have if fact stopped it. The report will alert providers in situations in which medication lists have not been kept up to date because once a patient stops warfarin prothrombin times will stop being drawn. When that patient is "overdue" for a prothrombin time, the physician or disease manager will update the chart to reflect stopping the warfarin.

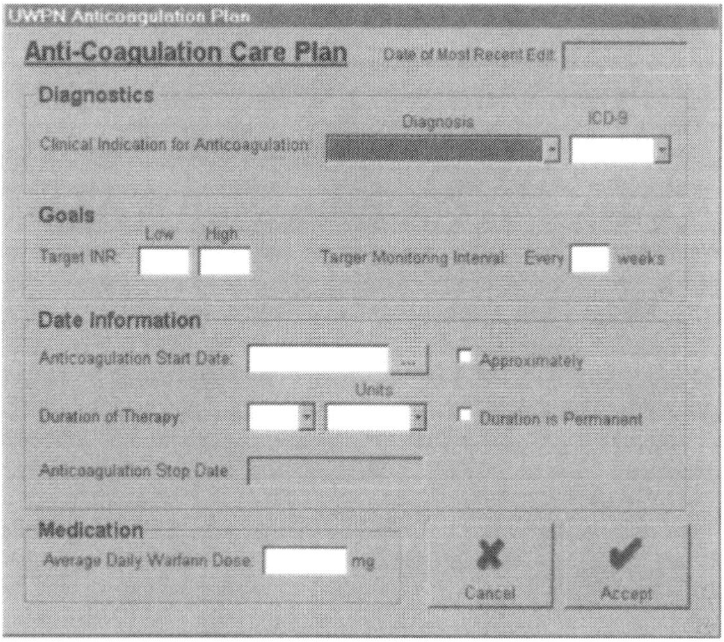

FIGURE 13.14. Data entry screen for recording individual patient care plan for anticoagulation.

Data Capture

The target INR range, duration of therapy, and frequency of monitoring will need to be entered for each patient who is on warfarin therapy. The program developers will create a data entry form, shown in Figure 13.14, which will be filled out for each patient on warfarin. The date and value for each prothrombin time are automatically put into the electronic medical record. These data are then compared to the target for that patient.

Developing the Report

The report will be designed as a tool for identifying warfarin patients in need of an INR test, a dose alteration, or treatment termination. It will also provide data for managing the population of patients on warfarin. As shown in Figure 13.15, the report to the anticoagulation manager shows the names of patients who are overdue for a prothrombin time, patients who are outside their target INR range, and patients whose charts show that they are still on warfarin after they were supposed to stop it.

Timeliness

The report will be run at the convenience of the anticoagulation manager. The longest interval between reports is to be a week, so automated reports will be generated each Monday. The report will be set up so that it can be run at any time.

Date 1/2/01 Patients on Warfarin:	Indication	Date Last	Target Interval	Last INR	Target INR	Therapy Duration	Start Date
Patient One	Cardioversion	12/18/00	2 weeks	1.8	2.0 – 3.0	4 weeks	11/23/00
Patient Two	Embolus	12/5/00	4 weeks	2.2	2.0 – 3.0	chronic	8/1/86
Patient Three	A Fib.	11/28/00	4 weeks	2.6	2.0 – 3.0	chronic	5/14/97
Patient Four	AVR	11/10/00	8 weeks	3.1	2.5 – 3.5	chronic	7/1/92
Patient Five	DVT	12/8/00	4 weeks	2.2	2.0 – 3.0	6 months	9/14/00
Patient Six	DVT	12/19/00	1 week	1.4	2.0 – 3.0	3 months	10/18/00
Patient Seven	A Fib.	12/1/00	4 weeks	2.5	2.0 – 3.0	chronic	4/15/91
Patient Eight	A Fib.	12/9/00	4 weeks	2.9	2.0 – 3.0	chronic	2/28/99
Patient Nine	DVT	12/3/00	4 weeks	2.4	2.0 – 3.0	3 months	9/18/00
Patient Ten	PE	12/17/00	2 weeks	2.0	2.0 – 3.0	chronic	11/14/94
Patient Eleven	CHF	12/8/00	4 weeks	3.1	2.0 – 3.0	chronic	6/4/97
Patient Twelve	AVR	12/8/00	4 weeks	2.3	2.5 – 3.5	chronic	2/12/98

FIGURE 13.15. A report of patients on warfarin showing patient in need of testing, dose adjustment and termination of therapy.

Specificity

When providers run the report, the default will be to show only their own patients. When the disease manager runs the report, she will be prompted to enter an individual provider, an entire clinic, or the network as a whole. The report will give both summary statistics and names of patients with specific, color-coded ways of identifying patients who are not meeting the targets that were individually set for them.

Future Directions

Healthcare data analysis is a growth industry, and the future will focus on how to use information to influence clinical decisions at the time they are made. New database systems will be developed merging administrative, financial, and clinical data, and more analyzable clinical data will be available directly from the provider-patient interface—including patient genetic information. On-line data analysis will become available, allowing real-time analysis of key information such as the result of a particular intervention. Voice recognition commands will be employed to pull data sets from vast data warehouses, which will store internal and external benchmarking statistics. Insurers, regulatory bodies, and accrediting agencies will make most clinical data analysis available to the public via the Internet, increasing the ability of individuals and organizations to access information about the type and quality of care provided, as well as increasing data security and confidentiality.

References

1. Austin C. *Information Systems for Hospital Administration.* Chicago, Health Administration Press, 1983.
2. Darby M. Managing data for quality improvement. *The Quality Letter* 1998 Jun; 2–9.

3. Nussbaum, GM, Ault SP. The best little data warehouse. *Journal of Healthcare Information Management,* 1998 Winter; 12(4): 82–87.
4. Hummel J. Building a computerized disease registry for chronic illness management of diabetes. *Clinical Diabetes* 2000;18:107–113.
5. Gilbreath E, Schilp JL. *Health Data Quest: How to Find and Use Data for Performance Improvement.* San Francisco, Jossey-Bass, 2000.
6. Brassard M. *The Memory Jogger.* Methuen, MA, Goal/QPC, 1988.
7. Carey RG, Lloyd, RC. *Measuring Quality Improvement in Healthcare: A Guide to Statistical Process Control Applications.* New York, Quality Resources, 1995.
8. Taplin SH, Barlow WE, Ludman E, MacLehos R, Meyer DM, Seger D, Herta D, Chin C, Curry S. Testing reminder and motivational telephone calls to increase screening mammography: A randomized study. *J Natl Cancer Inst* 2000 Feb 2;92(3):233–42.
9. Teich JM, Sittig DF, Kuperman GJ, Chueh HC, Zielstorff RD, Glaser JP. Components of the optimal ambulatory care computing environment. *Medinfo* 1998;9 Pt 2:1273–7.
10. Leape LL, Kabcenell AI, Gandhi TK, Carver P, Nolan TW, Berwick DM. Reducing adverse drug events: Lessons from a breakthrough series collaborative. *Jt Comm J Qual Improv* 2000 Jun;26(6):321–31.
11. Berwick DM. Eleven worthy aims for clinical leadership of health system reform, *JAMA* 1994 Sep 14;272(10):797–802.
12. Payne TH, Murphy GR, Salazar AA. How well does ICD9 represent phrases used in the medical record problem list? *Proc Annu Symp Comput Appl Med Care* 1992:654–7.
13. Guideline for perioperative cardiovascular evaluation for noncardiac surgery, *Circulation* 1996 Mar 15;93(6):1278–317.
14. Wagner EH, Austin BT, Von Korff M. Improving outcomes in chronic illness. *Manag Care Q* 1996 Spring;4(2):12–25.
15. Tiggelaar JM, Love DW, Pahl RC. Establishing a pharmacy clinic in a city-county health department. *Drug Intell Clin Pharm* 1984 May;18(5):415–6.

14
Telecommunications in Primary Care

DAVID MASUDA, M.D.

> *The grand irony of our times is that the era of computers is over. All the major con-*
> *sequences of stand-alone computers have already taken place. Computers have*
> *speeded up our lives a bit, and that's it. In contrast, all the most promising technolo-*
> *gies making their debut now are chiefly due to communication between computers—*
> *that is, to connections rather than to computations. And since communication is the*
> *basis of culture, fiddling at this level is indeed momentous.*[1]
>
> Kevin Kelly, 1997

Medicine and Healthcare: The Realities

It may seem odd to argue that "the era of computers is over," given the myriad and significant contributions of computer technology described in the preceding chapters. From electronic health records to clinical decision support, computers seem poised to transform medicine and healthcare in the next decade. The distinction remains valid, if subtle, however. The tools and services described to this point are rarely "stand-alone" computing. Practical informatics will be *connected* computing, and in this sense Kelly's predictions make sense. A PC in a physician's office will be linked to millions of other systems across the globe, able to retrieve data and information and knowledge from a diverse wealth and depth of resources. Momentous, indeed.

The Clinical Scenario

Reflecting on the clinical scenarios presented in prior chapters, we can develop a sense of the breadth and depth of tools and services that "functional informatics" can bring to primary care medicine. With the electronic medical record, clinical decision support, and clinical information systems (as well as other applications), computing technology has brought about dramatic change in the nature of medical practice, and it has the potential to bring about much more. Most expect that the pace of change will accelerate in the coming two decades.

These changes become even more significant when we consider the role that communications plays and will play in primary care. In the hypothetical case in Chapter 1—a patient with metastatic breast cancer who "fell through the cracks"—a nontrivial amount of information was created in the course of a busy clinical day. Prior to functional informatics, the tools to generate, store, transmit, exchange, and reuse information were quite limited. However when the newer informatics tools are applied, the process and outcomes of care can improve significantly. The case suggests that, to the clinician and to the patient, the overall value of information grows meaningfully when it is enhanced with informatics. It is arguable that value of the information grows exponentially when it can also be shared with all the various stakeholders in the healthcare process. This principle has been called Metcalfe's law:[2] the value of information rises exponentially relative to the number of nodes in a network. The common example is the fax machine. Not only were the first fax machines very expensive, they also had very limited value because there were so few between which information could be sent. As more and more fax machines became linked to the telecommunications network, the value of each machine rose exponentially. To optimally share and gain maximal value from information, it must be communicated.

"Connected" Clinical Scenarios

In Chapter 1 we considered the case of Alicia Jones, a young woman who succumbed to metastatic breast cancer. A less tragic alternative to her case was also presented, one that described the potential enhancement that "functional informatics" might have brought to her care—possibly averting an adverse outcome. In the alternative scenario, several computing applications were described. If we look more closely, we will recognize that in each case, the added value was not due to "stand-alone" computing, but to "connected" computing. To use his electronic medical record and clinical decision support tools, the family physician's desktop computer linked to his local area network. To retrieve and view the lab data and radiology images, his computer linked to a hospital wide area network. To find and use evidence-based medicine and library resources, his computer went out to the World Wide Web. To perform the billing functions and utilize workflow tools, his computer linked to an intranet and to the Internet. So in this scenario, both local and distant "connected" computing is crucial.

To broaden the perspective on functional telecommunications, we have to look beyond the connected computer. We must consider that "computers" will increasingly look less and less like the CPU-monitor-keyboard setup that now sits on our desk. The connected computing tools we use in the future will come in many shapes. They will be small, wearable, perhaps even implantable. Above all, they will be ubiquitous.

A few additional scenarios should demonstrate the changes that are coming.

• *The connected telephone*   A 26-year-old white male is involved in a MVA, sustaining multiple facial fractures, a hemothorax, and a femoral fracture. His emergent care requires timely and efficient coordination of several specialists—a general surgeon, an orthopedic surgeon, an oral surgeon, and a plastic surgeon. Historically this has meant often frustrating communication using multiple tools: face-to-face dialog, intercoms, telephones, and pagers. With functional telecommunications, each of these specialists carries a single device that plays all these roles. Nomadic computers, such as Web-enabled palm devices, with built-in wireless telephony, messaging, text and data display, multipoint conferencing, and global positioning systems will permit speedy collaborative decision making.

- *The connected television*   A 66-year-old healthy white male comes into the office concerned about a mole that has changed in size and color over the past 3 months. Unfortunately, the nearest dermatologist to this rural practice is 75 miles away. Moreover, there is a 3-week wait for an appointment in his office. With functional telecommunications the rural provider has two options—he can use a digital still camera to take several "snapshots" of the suspicious lesion, download them into his computer, and attach them to an e-mail message to a tele-dermatologist, and expect a teleconsult response in less than 24 hours. Alternatively, he can accompany his patient to the telehealth studio in his office and engage in a two-way interactive real-time videoconsultation with the teledermatologist. Not only does the patient receive a specialist's consultation the PCP receives a mini CME session on the workup of changing skin lesions. And no one had to leave town.
- *The connected researcher.*   A 68-year-old female patient with stage 3 lung cancer for whom traditional chemotherapy has failed would like to be considered for a new, still-experimental chemotherapeutic regimen she discovered on a Web search from her home. However, the only site currently approved and enrolling patients in this study protocol is an academic research center in South America. With functional telecommunications, the study designers in Peru are linked to a Web service that finds and connects them with willing experimental subjects around the globe. The protocols, treatments, and follow-up care can be provided by the patient's local physician and study data sent via the Web to the study center. Not only are patients able to gain access to care that otherwise might not be available, but the times to complete such complex studies are dramatically reduced.
- *The connected community*   In a small middle-western U.S. city of 250,000 people, a diverse group of community leaders have come together, increasingly concerned over the rising costs of healthcare and the inefficiencies and frustrations of healthcare delivery in both clinics and hospitals. Physicians, hospitals, patients, employers, schools, insurers, government agencies, and public health departments gather to discuss their individual needs, interests, and concerns. They also learn of the needs and interests of each of the other stakeholders. They begin to realize that they all face significant information deficits and that many of these deficits could be resolved if they could agree to share data and information. They agree to build a local community health information network—a CHIN—in which all the stakeholders share data and information.
- *The connected teacher*   The local general surgeon would like to add minimally invasive surgery to her current set of skills. The nearest academic center where she can learn this technique is 200 miles away, and the required training period is a month. However the Department of Surgery at the regional academic medical center is soon to go live with their new distance-learning surgery program. Using the incredibly high speeds and bandwidth of the next-generation Internet, they have been able to create and successfully test a "telepresence training program." After the surgeon completes a Web-based didactic program on the procedure at home in the evenings, the university ships to her a mobile virtual reality suite, consisting of a high-resolution camera and monitor, real-time two-way

audio and video connections, head-mounted displays on both ends, and roboti-
cally controlled endoscopic devices. As the local surgeon begins her first virtual
case, the expert at the university is able to oversee each maneuver. He can even
take control of the instruments should that be necessary—robotic surgery. After
completing the first case successfully, the local surgeon completes five more
under the guidance of her telementor and then is given certification of competence in the new procedure.

These hypothetical cases demonstrate not only the increasingly broad spectrum
of telecommunications channels and tools that can enhance the practice of primary care but also the multiplicity of parties that can benefit from information
sharing. It should be increasingly obvious that as more and more information is
shared among stakeholders, the overall value of the information to each increases.
If Kelly's assessment is accurate, primary care informatics will undergo fundamental change as it embraces the forms of evolving telecommunications.

Telecommunications: A Model

Medical textbooks describing technology suffer under Moore's law, named after
Gordon Moore, then chairman of Intel, who discovered in 1965[3] that computing
power (as measured by the number of transistors on a single CPU (Central Processing Unit)) doubles every 18 to 24 months. This law (which continues to hold
today) also means that any textbook written to describe the current state of technology arguably becomes only half-accurate 18 months after the publication date.
In an effort to overcome this limitation, we might consider an alternative—instead
of simply describing communications technology circa early 2001, we might construct a telecommunications model that will retain validity regardless of the
specifics of the new technology just over the horizon.

One such model could consider the communication of healthcare information
framed in three questions:

1. What information can be shared?
2. With whom might information be shared?
3. What technologies enable sharing, both now and in the future?

While some answers are self-evident, others are less so.

What Information Can Be Shared?

Clinical Information

As noted by Ketchell in Chapter 8, there are several types of information that primary care physicians require in daily practice. Paul Gorman has expanded on the
work of others to develop a valuable model of information types in patient care.[4]
This model encompasses the two intuitive types of information, patient data and
medical knowledge (Table 14.1). *Patient data* is defined as information unique to

TABLE 14.1 Clinical information types.

Type of information	Description	Examples	Sources
Patient data	Refers to a single person	Medical history Physical exam Lab and X-ray data	Patients, family Medical record
Medical knowledge	Generalizable to many persons	Original research Textbook descriptions Common knowledge	Journals Textbooks Consultants, colleagues
Logistic information	How to get the job done	Required forms Covered procedures	Local policy/procedure manuals Managed care organizations
Population statistics	Aggregate patient data	Recent patterns of illness Public health data Health plan data	Recent memory Public health departments
Social influences	How others get the job done	Local practice patterns	Discussion with colleagues

Source: Adapted from Borman PN. Information needs of physicians, *J Am Soc Inf Sci* 1995;46:729–736.

an individual and by example is the information in a patient's chart, such as the problem list, the history of present illness, the physical exam findings, laboratory and radiology reports, and consultant's reports. *Medical knowledge* describes information about how to practice medicine and is generalizable to all patients. Medical knowledge is generated from medical research and is typically contained in textbooks, journals, and, of course, physicians' heads. Generally speaking, medical knowledge is knowledge of how to diagnosis and treat illness and injury. When synthesized, the two information types enable the basic patient care process.

From the table, it is clear that day-to-day medical practice requires other types of information of no lesser importance. Gorman describes three additional types of information: logistic information, population statistics, and social influences. Logistic information is information on how to get the job done and may be unique to each practice and setting. Logistic information may be captured in the answers to such questions as "How do I order an MRI study for this patient?" and "Does this patient's insurance company require preauthorization for a referral to a specialist?" Population statistics is described as aggregated data about populations of patients and can be considered from both an epidemiologic and a managed care perspective. Epidemiologically, population statistics includes answers to questions such as "Does the apparent increased number of sore throats in the office this week suggest that we are in the midst of an outbreak of influenza?" From the care management perspective, one question could be "How can I get a list of all the eligible female patients in my practice who did *not* have a screening mammogram this past year?" Finally, social influences are the local norms and expectations about how medicine works. These are generated by clinicians, patients, families, and others in a community. Social influence information might include the answer to a question such as "How do I treat this patient for x when the patient's culture/nationality does not permit use of treatment y ?"

While medical knowledge and patient data are obvious forms of information in medical practice, the additional three types may be less so, but they are no less important. Moreover, it should also be clear that the sources of such information are not always the same as patient data (the medical record) and medical knowledge (textbooks and journals). The additional types of information may come from a wide variety of sources, including public health departments and other government sources, third-party payers and health plans, patients and family members, or colleagues (to name a few). But as often as not, these types of information are not easily available. Ideally, the newer telecommunications tools will begin to resolve some of these needs.

Two final points are important as we develop the healthcare information telecommunications model. First, it is important to realize that Gorman's work focuses on the categorization of clinical information needs. A successful and productive medical practice includes not only clinical work and workers but any number of nonclinical workers doing nonclinical work, as well. These people have similar information needs. Second, Gorman's model of information needs primarily defines information entering a medical practice. It should be clear that medical practices also generate considerable amounts of information and that there are many individuals and entities that consume this information (payers, patients, hospitals, and regulatory agencies, for example). Therefore, the direction of information flow is also very important to consider.

Returning once again to Kelly's observations, the telecommunications-enhanced medical practice will be one in which both clinical and nonclinical information are widely dispersed and received.

Nonclinical Information

Clearly, a large volume of information is generated moment to moment in a primary care practice that is used by nonclinicians. Interestingly, Gorman's model still holds. Obviously, patient data is generated, and it may include demographic information, insurance information, and employment information. Logistic information is also generated: how patient appointments are scheduled in any given practice, which insurance plans the practice accepts, how patients are instructed to call their providers. Social influence information is generated in the same way that patient-based social information comes into being; practices are social entities, and each may have varying social standards and variables. Population statistics are generated both through reporting reportable disease cases that come through the practice and by the various measures of quality (outcomes and process) and satisfaction that may be required of the practice by various health plans or accrediting agencies such as NCQA or by the practice's own internal quality improvement plans. Even medical knowledge can be generated as practices are involved in academic research in primary care practice.

Direction of Information Flow

In "communication," as the word is most commonly understood, information flows in two directions—both into and out from a medical practice. This bidirectional information flow also fits Gorman's model.

For example, when a patient is referred to a specialist, patient-specific information is communicated from the PCP to the specialist in the form of the patient's chart or chart summary, and the specialist's findings are sent to the PCP. Logistic information—the "business" of a medical practice—is communicated between PCP and insurance companies. The provider might ask the question "Does this patient's insurance company require pre-authorization for a referral to a specialist?" The insurer would ask, "What is the PCP's provider number and electronic billing address so that we can reimburse appropriately?" Social influences information is communicated by the PCP as contributions to the norms and standards of practice in their community. Population information is communicated in managed care environments as PCPs collect and analyze data and are accredited according to their performance in preventive care and population health improvement. Similarly, PCPs can contribute to population public health as they participate in mandated disease surveillance systems.

With Whom Might Information Be Shared?

Where does all the information generated by a medical practice go? Where does the information received come from? A surprising number of people and organizations have an interest in healthcare information. As we consider wider and wider circles of communication, the links become less obvious, but they are no less significant.

We can model information-sharing partners by the relationships they have with practices and by the functions they have in a practice. The partners who have direct relationships to the PCP or practice include the immediate partners in the healthcare process, such as clinic and hospital nurses, other physicians, and various mid-level providers. Similarly, the patients themselves and the patients' immediate families or friends are often intimately involved in a direct communication relationship. At a level somewhat more removed are *indirect* communication and information-sharing relationships. The list of partners in the indirect category may include the patient's insurer and employer. If the patient is of a younger age, the school system may be included. Depending on the nature of the patient's health conditions, public health entities and even law enforcement may be involved. Also on the list are professional medical societies, legal firms, and news agencies. As managed care changes the processes and business of care, regulators and accreditors (JCAHO, NCQA) are brought into the loop. From the business perspective, a wide range of vendors, suppliers, laboratories, and pharmacies may be involved.

As mentioned, a second model of conceptualizing information partners is by the function they play on the process. Some of the typical functions in a primary care practice include care provision (information sharing between physicians, nurses, hospitals, and complementary care providers), practice management (information sharing between payers, health plans, accrediting agencies, regulators, and vendors), and continuing education (information sharing between universities and professional societies).

What Technologies Enable Sharing, Both Now, and in the Future?

As we consider both a broad range of information types and a similarly broad range of information partners, we can begin to see the functional limitations of conventional telecommunications tools and services—how they hinder effective, efficient information sharing. We may also begin to develop an appreciation for new and innovative communications tools and services—those that are emerging today and those that are still beyond the horizon.

Modes of Telecommunications

Clearly, the 1990s saw tremendous growth and evolution in the modes of telecommunications that are available to medicine and healthcare. It is, of course, the electronic mode in which the majority of changes occurred and in which we see the greatest promise for revolutionary processes in medicine. The connection of computers through the Internet, providing e-mail, Web sites, and other products and services, is perhaps the most obvious example of this dramatic change.

Historic Telecommunications Channels

The ways physicians and other workers in medical practice have communicated historically are well-known, and those that have become universally adopted fulfill a clear need in an efficient, effective way. One way to classify currently used channels is following the concept of time: synchronous and asynchronous communication. Synchronous communication occurs when two or more people communicate contemporaneously. A conversation is the best example. Conversations can occur face to face, over a two-way radio or the telephone, even via smoke signals. Asynchronous communication occurs when the two (or more) conversants participate at different points in time. For example, a letter, a journal article, and a paper medical record are forms of asynchronous communication, as are faxes and pager messages. Communication channels can also be modeled from the perspective of mode. In primary care medicine the modes of communication have been primarily three types: face to face (conversations), paper-based (letters and documents), and electronic (phone calls and faxes.).

Arguably, conversations are the fundamental building block of communication, and over the centuries conversations have been both enhanced and altered as new technologies have changed both the time and mode of conversation. Beginning with spoken language and followed by the spoken word, the printed word, and now the digital word, new telecommunications technologies have continuously driven the evolution of communication. In our lifetimes, the telephone—effectively the first electronic healthcare communication tool—has had a tremendous impact. At a very basic level, the telephone engenders a fundamental change in communication—it vastly extends reach (in terms of both time and distance). With telephone-enhanced communication, information can be shared globally, at the speed of light. In addition, it has a very familiar user interface and is relatively inexpensive and highly reliable. In short, it is an indispensable tool in any medical practice. Related tools, such as pagers and fax machines, fulfill similar needs in slightly different niches.

All technology, in fact all communication, has both intended and unintended consequences. "Intended consequences may or may not happen, unintended consequences always do."[5] An exploration of telecommunications in primary care must also reflect on the problems and obstacles that arise. For example, face-to-face conversations are increasingly difficult to carry out when patient appointments grow ever shorter and clinic days grow ever longer. We are so deluged with paper-based communications that there is little time at the end of the day to read them all, much less generate well-considered letters and chart notes. And as irreplaceable as the telephone is, busy signals, telephone tag, and telemarketing nuisance calls increasingly frustrate the busy clinician. It is evident that best use of these tools requires an understanding of the trade-offs. Fortunately, functional telecommunications, enhanced with functional informatics, offers hope that new solutions, wisely adopted, will bring new value to healthcare.

Newer Electronic Telecommunications Channels

Before describing some of the newer applications of the electronic mode of communications, we should briefly explore the range of physical connections that can link healthcare providers and the range of information devices that lie at either end of these connections. An inherent part of this discussion are the enabling technologies and the standards that make them interoperable.

Physical Connections

Electronic telecommunications, for the most part, still require some sort of "wire" to link people together. A major revolution of the last decade has been the relatively rapid shift from copper wire to fiber-optic cable. Copper wire is the basis for a number of telecommunications channels, including POTS (plain old telephone service), cable television, and computer network cables. One of the inherent limitations of copper wire is that there is a finite limit on the amount of electronic digital information that can be passed through it. This concept of information volume per unit of time, often called "bandwidth," is a significant issue for telecommunications. The amount of information carried in a typical analog voice telephone call is relatively small, so copper telephone wire is perfectly sufficient to handle voice telephony. However, as more and more information becomes digital, the volume of information exceeds the ability of copper wire to transmit at reasonable speeds. Anyone who has recently experienced accessing the Internet with an older, slower modem (28.8 bps, for example) understands this limitation. Although some newer protocols, such as ADSL, can increase the speed traveling through copper wires, the future is far more likely to lie in replacing copper wire entirely with fiber optics. Simply, the process is one of transforming electrical signals in copper wire to pulses of light that travel through extremely small glass fibers. The volume of information that can be carried in glass fibers is exponentially larger than the amount of information that can be carried in copper wires of similar dimension. In addition, fiber is cheaper and more reliable. Fiber is relatively more expensive, however, because there is already such a large installed base of copper, and replacing it with fiber will take time. This is known as the "last mile" problem—getting fiber all the way to the primary care office—and it probably will not happen in the near future.

More recently, connectivity without wires has come to the fore. Often known as "wireless," this physical connection uses various spectra of radio and microwaves to transmit information. The more commonly known uses include pagers and telephones ("cellular" or "digital" services). The advantages of wireless connectivity are obvious. The absence of a physical connection makes any wireless information device entirely mobile, as long as it can be carried. Therefore wireless permits true "ubiquitous connectivity." The primary disadvantage of wireless has been somewhat less consistent signals, prone to interference, and slower speeds of communication (often no better than slower modem connections). Current wireless transmission bandwidth is more than adequate for voice transmission. By 2004, we can expect to see significant advances in wireless transmission speeds, a development that will transform wireless communications. The other primary limitation to wireless communication is incomplete coverage. In urban environments wireless services are extensively available but in rural parts of the country, availability can be significantly less (and at the same time cost more). Coverage is likely to be resolved through two developments, expansion of existing land-based wireless transmitting stations and developments in two-way satellite wireless transmission.

One last physical connection requires mention. As use of the Internet has grown exponentially, the need for an even faster global network has become clear. At the same time, the need for greater bandwidth to enable advanced applications has become clear. These forces have driven the development of a second-generation Internet. Internet2 is a joint venture of industry, the federal government, and academic institutions to develop a very high-speed backbone network across the United States. As this network becomes more widely available, the range of information types that can be communicated will increase significantly.

Networks

Whether channels are copper, fiber, or wireless, they can be arranged and connected in a number of ways. An in-depth discussion of networking topology is beyond the scope of this chapter, but a very brief summary of networking concepts may be helpful. In essence, networks can be characterized as a function of size and reach. A network can be as simple as two office computers linked together (often called a peer-to-peer network). When two or more computers are linked locally, within a clinic or hospital, the connection is called a local area network. Wide area networks generally encompass a larger geographic distribution, perhaps several clinics surrounding a central hospital site. A metropolitan area network is a large number of computers and computer peripherals linked in metropolitan urban area.

Regardless of the topology of networks, they have in common some set of shared protocols that define the nature of the information signals that are exchanged between devices on the network. A large number of protocols are in use today, the most significant of which is called TCP/IP. TCP/IP is the protocol that supports the Internet and allows every computer connected to the Internet to communicate with other computers and other information devices. Readers interested in additional information might access on-line resources.[6,7]

Newer Telecommunications Tools

Whether the communications channel is copper, fiber optic, or wireless, at either end of the communication linkage must be some sort of information device that can send, receive, and translate data and information. The range of information devices currently in common use are telephones, fax machines, and pagers. Radio and television might also be included in the list. There are also commonly used clinical devices that communicate—remote telemetry sensors, programmable pacemakers, and the like. The functions these tools perform are fairly straightforward and well understood. Perhaps the most obvious of the newer communications tools is the desktop computer. Whether it is e-mailing or Web browsing, this information device clearly benefits greatly from connectivity. Moreover, the connected computer increases the typical range of information that is communicated. No longer are we talking about text or data or voice or images; all these modalities are combined in one information device. The functions of computers are covered elsewhere in this book. We now turn our attention to other information devices and describe a number of directions in which information devices are likely to evolve.

Miniaturization, Hybridization, and Independence

In the coming decade we will see three significant trends affect all information devices—miniaturization, hybridization, and independence. In other words, information devices will get smaller, they will provide more and more functions (functions that heretofore have required multiple devices), and they will no longer need to be physically connected through a wire or cable. Cellular phones are the prototypical example. The first generation of cellular phones were extremely bulky, involving not only a handset but also a small briefcase for the battery and transmission equipment. Miniaturization progressed at a rapid rate—in the year

2000 the first truly functional wristwatch wireless telephone became commercially available, fulfilling the technology expectation laid out in the *Dick Tracy* cartoon decades ago.

In addition to progressive miniaturization, the range of functionality available on wireless telephones is increasing. The most obvious example is the marriage of wireless telephones with personal digital assistants (PDA). PDAs, alternatively known as palmtop computers, represent a larger concept of nomadic computing—the notion that the computer no longer needs to be connected by power cord or telephone/Ethernet cable. The first generation of palmtop devices were simple four-function machines. The functions included a personal calendar, an address book, a "to do" list, and a notepad. A basic arithmetical calculator was also included which, interestingly enough, represents an earlier form of hybridization—merging the calculator with a personal digital assistant. Current generations of PDAs include color as opposed to grayscale displays and higher resolution screens, allowing for display of more detailed text and images. Some palm devices include more functionality, in effect the range of tools available on a desktop computer, such as word processing, spreadsheets, and databases. There is a large and rapidly growing market for medical tools and software that take advantage of the database potential of palmtop devices. Typical examples are databases of drug dosages, E and M coding for office billing, and rudimentary electronic medical records that allow both entry and retrieval of data. As palm devices are merged with wireless telephones, these devices are becoming a portal to the Internet; e-mail and Web-browsing capabilities are appearing on newer generations of these tools. In short, it is very likely that within the next decade we will have the ability to carry on our belt or in our briefcase or purse a device that will function as a wireless video telephone, pager, radio, personal assistant, e-mail and Web browser, electronic medical record, and music player.

Applied Telecommunications in Primary Care

In the future of primary care medicine, perhaps more important than the tools for telecommunications will be the ways in which we apply electronic devices and networks to the processes of healthcare. To conclude this chapter we explore three of the arguably most significant developments: telemedicine, clinical e-mail, and community health information networks:

Telemedicine and Telehealth

One of the difficulties in discussing telemedicine is that a single commonly held definition of the term does not exist. Narrowly defined, telemedicine is the use of two-way interactive videoconferencing that enables a primary care provider and a patient to interact with a remote consulting specialist in, for example, orthopedics or psychiatry or cardiology. Alternative narrower definitions include the existing models of teleradiology and telepathology. It is valuable to consider telemedicine in a broader perspective. Telemedicine has been defined as "rapid access to shared and remote medical expertise by means of telecommunications and information technologies, no matter where the patient or relevant information is located."[8] Reid proposes another definition: the use of telecommunications technology to exchange information that provides access to healthcare across time, social, and cultural barriers.[9] Coiera provides a similar definition: "The essence of telemedicine is the exchange of information at a distance, whether that information is voice, an image, elements of the medical record, or commands to a surgical robot. It seems reasonable to think of telemedicine as the remote communication of information to facilitate clinical care."[10] But to fully understand the significance of telemedicine, the definition should also capture the notion that telecommunications will transform the very nature of medicine and healthcare. This transformation role will include physicians, the economics and markets of medicine, and patients as consumers. Bauer offers such a definition: "Telemedicine is the combined use of telecommunications and computer technologies to improve efficiency and effectiveness of health care services by liberating caregivers from traditional constraints of place and time by empowering consumers to make informed choices in a competitive marketplace."[11] In this sense, telemedicine may come to include communications and connectivity in which physicians play a tangential role or, in some cases, no role in all, clearly a significant transformation.

While the computing revolution seems to have become significant only in the last 10 to 20 years, telemedicine has been in existence for at least four decades. In fact, it is arguable that the very first instance of telemedicine took place in 1876 as Alexander Graham Bell spoke the now famous words "Mr. Watson, come here. I want to see you" into his new invention, the telephone.[12] His choice of words is alleged to have been a request for medical attention: Bell had just spilled battery acid on his hands. Modern telemedicine had its origins in the 1960s when the U.S. Department of Defense began to utilize satellite linkages to connect care providers on the U.S. mainland with military troops either at sea or in remote battlefield locations. Due to the costs and highly technical aspects of this form of telemedicine, the technology did not become widely adopted, and in fact by the 1980s most preexisting telemedicine programs had disappeared.

With the advent of inexpensive, powerful computers and then the Internet and the Web, a resurgence of interest in telemedicine applications, tools, and services took place in the 1990s. As with earlier experiments and programs, many of the initial approaches were two-way real-time interactive videoconferencing applications. Newer teledevices enhanced interactive video—digital stethoscopes, ophthalmoscopes, and otoscopes enabled the video consultation to more closely simulate an in-person visit. Shortly thereafter, the range of applications began to grow. For example, in addition to televideo, the transmission of still images has become valuable. Beginning with teleradiology and telepathology (essentially transmission of X rays and pathology slides in a digital format), this application has grown to include still images of many types. Digital photographs of skin lesions enables the practice of teledermatology, and digital representations of 12-lead ECGs enables telecardiology.

Still image transmission applications as a group, are known as "store-and-forward" telemedicine. This concept encompasses two components. The first is that telemedicine in this setting does not require providers at either end of the communication to be on line simultaneously. For example, a primary care provider who has a patient in the office with a potentially suspicious solitary skin lesion can now take a series of digital photographs of the lesion and attach them to an e-mail message to a remote dermatologist, with the expectation that the dermatologist will sometime in the next 12 to 24 hours review the images and return an e-mail consultation. The two-way interactive videoconferencing consultation is a form of synchronous communication; store-and-forward telemedicine can be considered asynchronous. Defining telemedicine as transmission of still images as well as video images begins to capture the broad definitions earlier in this section. In this sense, any form of data or information that enhances the healthcare process is in the realm of telemedicine.

One type of data transmission that may take telemedicine even closer to the broad definition would be communicating human physical actions over a distance. This would, of course, allow for "telesurgery." Telepresence could certainly enhance aspects of surgery. It would enable the process of mentoring and training of surgeons in new procedures and techniques. The actual performance of surgery via robotic devices that are guided by surgeons at some distance will probably become more frequent over time. There are several potential uses of telesurgery, many of which fall outside the realm of "usual" primary care. These include situations in which the surgeon is not available (remote or frontier areas and outer space), situations when the patient is in a hazardous environment (a battlefield or the scene of a nuclear accident), and situations where there is a practical barrier (patients with highly communicable diseases).[13]

In one sense, minimally invasive surgery and laparoscopic surgery are the earliest forms of telesurgery and robotics. Placing the surgeon's fingers even slightly distant from the scalpel and suture presages the development of digital robotics where a surgeon with electronic tools and communications will manipulate the blade from a great distance. One of the biggest remaining obstacles is the haptic device—a robotic tool that transmits the tactile sensations surgeons trust in standard surgery to determine precision of movement.

In the same way that the range of medical services that may be delivered via telemedicine is growing, the users of telemedicine must also be considered in a larger context. Just as one patient and one primary care provider in the clinic can communicate over a distance with one consulting specialist, telemedicine linkages can be built between providers and patients in many locations, not only clinics and hospitals but also nursing homes, public health agencies, educational facilities, prisons, shopping malls, and, of course, private homes. Although the entire range of clinical services can be delivered to diverse locales; most common would be radiology, pathology, cardiology, dermatology, psychiatry, and orthopedics.

As with the introduction of any new technology into medicine and healthcare, telemedicine brings with it both benefits and burdens. The potential benefits that telemedicine will bring include cost reduction by reducing the number of unnecessary consultations; reduction of inconvenience by allowing patients to remain in their own locale and "virtually" bringing the specialist to the patient; reduction of the professional isolation experienced by rural providers by videoconferencing, which provides not only care delivery but also education; and enhancement of standardized, evidence-based care by more frequent and more timely communication between specialists and primary care providers.

Telemedicine means potential burdens, as well. Currently, videoconferencing is still a technically limited interaction. Videoconferences are likely to be frustrating due to telecommunications inconsistencies. Videoconferences involving three people (the patient, the local provider, and the remote specialist) introduces a new examination room dynamic: both care provision and education occur, which can be time consuming. There are a number of legal issues, including state medical licensure (Where is the "practice" of medicine taking place—where the patient resides or where the specialist resides?) and liability (Is the standard of care for telemedicine the same as or different from that of in-person medicine?). Reimbursement policies are unsettled. And there are the large number of questions about confidentiality, privacy, and security as personal health data and information are communicated across time and distance.

In addition, telemedicine is only beginning to undergo rigorous clinical quality evaluation studies. There is relatively little clear and compelling data on the impact of telemedicine for healthcare delivery quality or cost. This limitation is compounded by the difficulty of evaluating a technology that is changing rapidly. On the other hand, there seems to be fairly clear evidence that both patient and provider satisfaction with applied telemedicine projects is high. It is probably only a matter of time before we obtain better evidence as to what constitutes a high-quality and quickly effective telemedicine intervention. This will occur because of two factors. Technological innovation will continue at a rapid rate and the practice of medicine itself will evolve rapidly as we begin to better understand how telemedicine communications technology can best be put to use on a regular basis in the practice of medicine. In short, we can expect that the concept of telemedicine as a separate entity in healthcare delivery will eventually fade away as it becomes part and parcel of daily activity. In the broadest definition of all, all medicine will be, in effect, telemedicine.

Clinical E-mail

If the broad definition of telemedicine is a wide range of information exchange across time and place, a very significant subset is e-mail linking physicians to each other and to their patients. The current use of clinical e-mail by primary care providers varies widely. Some practices have flatly refused to adopt this technology; other practices use it widely although indiscriminately; some practices have adopted clinical e-mail in a systematic and formal way. It is likely that over the next decade, the use of clinical e-mail will grow dramatically and will become at least an equally if not more valuable and mandatory tool for communicating with other clinicians and with patients than the telephone.

E-mail is a unique method of communication. Lying somewhere between the written and the spoken word, it has advantages of both. Since it is delivered far more quickly than letters, it has a higher level of spontaneity and timeliness. It is not instantaneous, as is a verbal conversation, so it allows for some period of reflection and composition of thought before replying. It eliminates the time waste of telephone tag and at the same time precludes the interruption of an incoming phone call or page (another example of asynchronous communication). Moreover, it is self-documenting—in almost every instance it automatically becomes a part of the permanent medical record. Advanced clinical e-mail systems permit templated messages—a significant number of patient requests for information are of a similar nature, so "canned" replies can be used effectively, and can be enhanced by the addition of personalized information. Similarly, e-mail can point patients toward additional information resources such as Web pages and people within an organization to whom a phone call or another e-mail message can be directed. It is not surprising, given these distinct capabilities, that patients are increasingly demanding that their physicians and other care providers communicate with them by e-mail. This demand will undoubtedly grow rapidly over the next few years.

As with telemedicine, there are a number of potential obstacles to more widespread use of clinical e-mail, both real and perceived. Perhaps the largest issue, one that has both real and perceived aspects, is that of the confidentiality, security, and privacy of a clinical e-mail exchange. There is a very high level of concern regarding the risks of inadvertent exposure of medical information via e-mail abuse or misuse on the part of both providers and patients. Although there are many possibilities for abusing patients' personal information, such as misaddressing or misrouting messages, intercepting messages, or misusing messages by clinical office personnel patient family members or patient employers, fotunately there are also technological solutions to these issues, including encryption and secure networks. In addition, organizational models help employees in a practice better understand the importance of confidentiality and security and provide organizational policies and procedures that enhance protection.

Another obstacle is the concern that communicating with patients via e-mail will increase exposure to medical liability. While there is some small risk that this will happen, it is more likely that clinical e-mail will provide protection in liability cases. As noted, e-mail has powerful self-documenting properties. Also, if a practice develops a well-considered and rational approach to the use of e-mail, including written policies and procedures, the risk of liability can be significantly reduced.

Certainly the introduction of clinical e-mail into a practice introduces a potential for workflow disruption. There is a common perception that allowing patients to exchange e-mail with providers will add dramatically to the already constrained physician time in a busy practice because of both a large number of incoming messages from patients and individual messages that are voluminous. In actual practice, neither problem seems to be common. The number of patients in a practice who abuse e-mail tends to be fairly small, and with proper instruction

TABLE 14.2 American Medical Informatics Association's guidelines for clinical use of electronic mail with patients.

Establish turnaround time for messages. Do not use e-mail for urgent matters.

Inform patients about privacy issues. Patients should know who besides addressee processes messages, both during addressee's usual business hours and during addressee's vacation or illness. That message is to be included as part of the medical record.

Establish types of transactions (prescription refill, appointment scheduling, etc.) and sensitivity of subject matter (HIV, mental health, etc.) permitted over e-mail.

Instruct patients to put category of transaction in subject line of message for filtering: "prescription," "appointment," "medical advice," "billing question."

Request that patients put their name and patient identification number in the body of the message.

Configure automatic reply to acknowledge receipt of messages.

Print all messages, with replies and confirmation of receipt, and place in patient's paper chart.

Send a new message to inform patient of completion of request.

Request that patients use autoreply feature to acknowledge reading provider's message.

Maintain a mailing list of patients, but do not send group mailings where recipients are visible to each other. Use blind copy feature in software.

Avoid anger, sarcasm, harsh criticism, and libelous references to third parties in messages.

the great majority of patients can use this tool both effectively and responsibly. In fact, expeditious use of e-mail can mitigate a number of other common workflow complaints in a practice. For example, e-mail communication can replace a significant number of phone calls both generated and received by the physician. In the former, physicians are freed from playing telephone tag. In the latter, they are freed from unexpected interruptions.

As with any new procedure or clinical process in a medical practice, understanding the risks and benefits is important, and it is a good idea to formulate official policies around new procedures and processes. The American Medical Informatics Association has published a widely accepted set of guidelines for the clinical use of electronic mail with patients;[14]—they are summarized in Table 14.2.

Community Health Information Networks (CHINs)

It seems reasonable to conclude our discussion of telecommunications and primary care with an exploration of community health information networks (CHINs). Although CHINS have experienced slower and less consistent growth than either telemedicine or clinical e-mail, they embody a concept that not only summarizes the ideas in this chapter but can provide a "big picture" way of thinking about primary care telecommunications.

A community health information network is a collection of individuals and organizations in a community who share an interest or stake in healthcare and believe that everyone in the healthcare process benefits when information is shared and communicated freely. The primary care practice is probably the simplest form of community health information network. Recalling the broad range of types of information generated and received in a primary care practice and understanding the types of personnel in a clinical practice, it is not a large stretch to state that any communications technology that allows for rapid and effective exchange of information within a practice will increase efficiency, quality, and satisfaction. The communication tools described in this chapter and the other informatics tools described in the preceding chapters all play various roles in information exchange.

Expanding this model to the next layer of information partners, a medical practice interacts with local specialist practices, the local hospital, and the various insurance companies and payers that provide coverage for the patients. Fairly robust communications channels may already exist with some of the layers, such as the insurance companies and payers, but the communication channels to other offices and the local hospital may be less robust. At the CHIN level is *any* individual or organization that has an interest in healthcare. The list can be lengthy and might include patients, schools, employers, libraries, public health departments, financial institutions, law enforcement organizations, and so on. Although the information that these groups may benefit from may be different in both scope and depth, it should be clear that any communications tools or services that enhance the transfer of the information has the potential to benefit all the involved parties.

The Hartford Foundation developed a formal definition for CHINs in 1994: "A community health management information system collects and disseminates healthcare-related data and analyses to meet a wide range of needs, building information resources throughout the community."[15] The term "community" in this definition has two meanings—the geographic entity of the network and the notion that such an entity can provide societal value. An alternative definition reads, "A community health information network is an innovative combination of services, products, and technology that enables organizations to exchange clinical, financial, and administrative information electronically with other designated organizations. The role of a CHIN is to enhance the efficiency and delivery of health care by allowing electronic exchange of information among health-care entities."[16] This definition captures the concept that a CHIN can involve a large number of people in other organizations than those that are involved in the direct provision of care. This developing model of the community health information network suggests that the primary care practice will increasingly become part of a larger healthcare community team. Just as primary care has evolved from the paternalistic model of the practice of medicine to one of shared decision making, the concept of CHINs suggests that all practices, even those that have previously been "informationally isolated," will increasingly participate in larger circles of information sharing.

The drivers behind the development of CHINs parallel the drivers of innovation in healthcare in general. They include escalating healthcare costs, an increasing concern for standardization and quality in healthcare, a growing understanding within healthcare that other industries such as banking and manufacturing have realized significant economic and quality improvements by embracing the concept of information sharing, and the shift of economic risk from payers to providers. Similarly, the enablers of CHINs include the increasing availability of powerful and affordable information and communications technology as well as the standards inherent in the Internet and the World Wide Web.

In recent years, approximately 500 CHINS (of various related types) have sprung up across the country. Many are in the early stages of development. The range of community organizations that are involved is different in each case, as are the reasons for which the CHINs have been formed. These reasons may include community service, research, pure care delivery, or competitive advantage. A number of different business models, organizational models, and ownership and control models have evolved as well.

The future of CHINs may be less clear than that of clinical e-mail or telemedicine—it will be necessary for these networks bring true value to the communities they serve. CHINs will also probably take several different forms, depending on the nature of the communities in which they arise. It seems likely that in many areas CHINs may develop only partially and involve only some of the healthcare constituents. Nevertheless, it is valuable for primary care clinicians to consider CHINs as a model that captures the significance of telecommunications and its potential.

Summary

Today we are witnessing the early, turbulent days of a revolution as significant as any other human history. A new medium of human communication is emerging, one that may prove to surpass all previous revolutions—the printing press, the telephone, the television—in its impact on our economic and social life. The computer is expanding from a tool for information management to a tool for communications. Interactive multimedia and the so-called information highway, and its exemplar the Internet, are enabling a new economy based on the networking of human intelligence. In this digital economy, individuals and enterprises create wealth by applying knowledge, networked human intelligence, and effort to manufacturing, agriculture, and services. In the digital frontier of this economy, the players, dynamics, rules, and requirements for survival and success are all changing.[17]

Don Tapscott, 1996

If Tapscott's predictions are accurate, the practice of primary care in the digital economy will undergo tremendous evolution in the next two decades. Computing and communication technologies will drive significant and dramatic change for "the players, dynamics, rules, and requirements" of medicine and healthcare. No community, provider, or practice will be immune, and the primary care in the year 2020 will undoubtedly be in some ways unrecognizable. As we utilize the computers sitting on our desks (or laps) and the digital wireless phones hanging from our belts, we may be able to envision medical practice in the next five years as information devices all interconnected through wireless communications, all exchanging a variety of information types, all informing a variety of healthcare constituents, but the vision of the future is far less clear. In many ways it will be better, in some ways it may be worse, depending on your point of view. Without doubt it will be different.

It is tempting to consider this rapid change as frightening and disorienting at best and detrimental to medicine and healthcare at worst. Regardless of one's perspective, it is safe to say that it is inevitable. With luck, the concepts in this chapter will aid primary care practitioners in developing a sense of the coming change and embracing the change so that the year 2020 will provide even more rewards than are present today.

When you think of the Internet, don't think of Mack truck full of widgets destined for distributorships, whizzing by countless billboards.
  Think of a table for two . . .

@man

References

1. http://www.wired.com/wired/archive/5.09/newrules.html
2. *Forbes ASAP,* September 13, 1993.
3. http://www.intel.com/intel/museum/25anniv/hof/moore.htm
4. Gorman PN. Information needs of physicians. *J Am Soc Inf Sci* 1995;46: 729–736.
5. Dee Hock, "The Birth of the Chaordic Century: Out of the Control and Into Order" (paper presented at the Extension National Leadership Conference, Washington, DC, 11 March 1996). http://www.fs.fed.us/im/philos/chaordic.htm
6. http://www.n-link.com/solutions/networking/
7. http://www.rad.com/networks/1997/nettut/main.html
8. CEC DG XIII. *Research and Technology Development on Telematics Systems in Health Care.* Annual technical report on RTD in health care. Brussels, AIM, 1993.
9. Reid J. *A Telemedicine Primer: Understanding the Issues.* Billings, MT, Innovative Medical Communication, 1996, p. 34.
10. Coiera, E. *Guide to Medical Informatics, the Internet and Telemedicine.* London, Chapman and Hall Medical, 1997, p. 224.
11. Bauer J. *Telemedicine and the Reinvention of Health Care.* New York; McGraw-Hill, 1999, p. 8.
12. http://memory.loc.gov/ammem/bellhtml/bell1.html
13. Stanberry B. *Telemedicine: Barriers and opportunities in the 21st century, J Int Med* 2000;247:615–28.
14. http://www.amia.org/pubs/other/email__guidelines.html
15. Dowling, A. *Community Health Information Networks.* New York, Springer-Verlag, 1996, p. 1.
16. Nutkis D, Golub R. Community health information networks: Pulse. Ernst & Young LLP, Spring 1995, pp. 11–15.
17. Tapscott D. *The Digital Economy.* New York, McGraw-Hill, 1996.

Index

.

30443391R00140